A Leader's Manual

For Dementia Care-Partner Support Groups

Edward G. Shaw M.D., M.A.

Alan D. Wolfelt Ph.D., C.T.

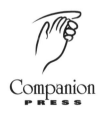

Companion
PRESS

An imprint of the Center for Loss and Life Transition
Fort Collins, Colorado

Companion Press is an imprint of the Center for Loss and Life Transition, 3735 Broken Bow Road, Fort Collins, Colorado 80526.

Companion Press books may be purchased in bulk for sales promotions, premiums, and fundraisers. Please contact the publisher at (970) 226-6050 or www.centerforloss.com for more information.

25 24 23 22 21 20   6 5 4 3 2 1

ISBN: 978-1-61722-293-1

Contents

INTRODUCTION 1
A word about *The Dementia Care-Partner's Workbook* 2
Why dementia care-partner support groups are important 4
The eight central needs of dementia care partners 6

BEFORE YOU BEGIN A SUPPORT GROUP 7
Deciding on a support-group leader 7
Needs assessment 8
Group format 9
Choosing a place and time of day to meet 11
Setting the number of members 11
Deciding on the number of lessons and frequency
and length of meetings 12
Recruiting and screening group members 13
Strategies to publicize the group 13
Establishing ground rules 16
Baseline and end-of-group assessments 16

BASIC SKILLS OF THE SUPPORT-GROUP LEADER 19
Responsibilities of the support-group leader 19
Qualities of the support-group leader 21
Defining leadership style 25

Basic counseling skills of the support-group leader 26

The nature and art of companioning 31

SUPPORT GROUP BASICS 33

Basic needs of support group members 33

The five developmental phases of a support group.................. 34

    Phase One (forming): Warm-up and establishing
group purpose and limits 34

    Phase Two (storming): Tentative self-disclosure
and exploring group boundaries................................ 36

    Phase Three (norming): In-depth self-exploration
and confronting the realities of caregiving 37

    Phase Four (working): Commitment
to healing and growth 38

    Phase Five (closing): Preparation for and
leaving the group 40

Challenges in the group... 42

    Lack of leader preparation and/or training 42

    Discrepancies between group members'
expectations and leader's expectations......................... 42

    Challenging members 43

Determining when a group member needs individual
counseling and asking a group member to leave the group 50

When the group just doesn't seem to be going well
and you're not sure why 52

    The leaders aren't doing their job well or
don't work well together.. 52

    The members don't mix well together......................... 52

When a group member or their loved one with dementia dies...... 53

MEETING PLANS FOR LESSONS ONE THROUGH TEN OF
THE DEMENTIA CARE-PARTNER'S WORKBOOK 55

A few words about members doing homework 56

Anatomy of a meeting plan 56

    If you plan to do baseline and end-of-group assessments 56

    Before the group begins 57

    Before group ("warmup") 57

    Opening the group 58

    Mindfulness Moment 58

    Check-in 59

    Education 60

    Discussion 60

    Preview of next meeting and homework 61

    Mindfulness Moment 61

    Closing 61

    After group ("afterburn") 62

    Leader and co-leader decompression time 62

MEETING ONE: Telling Your Story from the Beginning 63

MEETING TWO: Basics of Alzheimer's
Disease and Other Dementias 69

MEETING THREE: Brain Structure and Function,
Activities of Daily Living, and Dementia Stages 73

MEETING FOUR: Adapting to Changing Relationships 77

MEETING FIVE: Coping with Grief and Loss 81

MEETING SIX: Stress and Self-Care 85

MEETING SEVEN: Getting More Help and
Transitioning Care 89

MEETING EIGHT: Legal, Financial, and End-of-Life Issues 93

MEETING NINE: Existential and Spiritual Questions 97

MEETING TEN: Retelling Your Story Starting Today 101

APPENDICES 105

Appendix 1: Support Group Ground Rules 107

Appendix 2: Zarit Caregiver Burden Scale 109

Appendix 3: Geriatric Depression Scale
and Geriatric Anxiety Scale 113

Appendix 4: Support Group Leader's Overview..................... 117

Appendix 5: The Eight Central Needs
of Dementia Care Partners... 127

Appendix 6: Symptoms of the Four Most
Common Forms of Dementia...................................... 129

Appendix 7: Understanding Our Emotions Exercise................ 133

Appendix 8: Activities of Daily Living and
the Stages of Dementia 135

Appendix 9: Wellness Wheel and Wellness Plan 141

Appendix 10: Support-Group Participant Evaluation Form 145

Appendix 11: Resource for Support Group Members............... 151

Appendix 12: Certificate of Dementia
Care-Partner Support Group Participation 155

SELECTED REFERENCES 157

FEEDBACK 159

ABOUT THE AUTHORS... 161

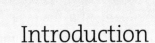

Introduction

Welcome, support-group leaders!

A Leader's Manual for Dementia Care-Partner Support Groups is to help you get started with and run a support group for dementia care partners in conjunction with *The Dementia Care-Partner's Workbook*. The comprehensive contents cover a variety of important topics that will allow you to plan and run a support group for dementia care partners. I am honored to have my friend and colleague Dr. Alan Wolfelt, a world-renowned grief counselor and author, as a co-author on this work. A veteran of writing grief support-group leader's manuals, Alan provided many of the thoughts and ideas you'll find herein. Whether you are a mental-health, medical, or other healthcare professional in the aging and dementia space, or a lay leader with the heart to lead a support group, it is my sincere hope that *The Dementia Care-Partner's Workbook* and this accompanying leader's manual will provide the resources necessary for you to minister to some of the now 18 million-plus care partners of a loved one with Alzheimer's disease or another form of dementia.

Please note that to use the ten-meeting plan, each of your group members will need to purchase a copy of *The Dementia Care-Partner's Workbook*. They are available through the Center for Loss website: www.centerforloss.com.

I hold you and those you will be helping in my thoughts and prayers. Dementia care partners often feel a great sense of isolation and loneliness, that no one else can understand the journey they are on. Being companioned by you, in a safe place where they can learn and understand more about dementia, the most feared of all human diseases, and receive compassion, affirmation, and hope, is truly a gift. Even on this journey down the path not chosen, thanks to you they will find comfort, companionship, and encouragement that tomorrow can be even better than today.

With warmth and blessings,

Edward G. Shaw, M.D., M.A.
Founder and former Director, Memory Counseling Program,
Wake Forest Baptist Health, Winston-Salem, NC
Founder, Empath Education

A WORD ABOUT *THE DEMENTIA CARE-PARTNER'S WORKBOOK*

The Dementia Care-Partner's Workbook was created as a flexible resource to provide understanding, education, and hope to care partners of those diagnosed with Alzheimer's disease or another form of dementia in either a support-group setting or as a self-study guide. Support groups are the backbone of the Memory Counseling Program I founded for dementia care partners at Wake Forest Baptist Health. Although many care partners initially feel hesitant to join a support group, our members feel an immediate sense of camaraderie and community with the very first meeting, relieved that someone else finally understands what they're going through. They consistently rate the program, curriculum, and group leaders very highly, and by the group's end, they also report greater knowledge about dementia and enhanced coping skills.

Our support-group program has two components: an initial ten-week classroom experience, corresponding to the ten lessons in *The*

Dementia Care-Partner's Workbook, followed by monthly maintenance groups. The classroom portion, offered three or four times yearly, is led by one or two counselors for groups of eight to 16 people who stay together for ten consecutive weekly meetings that are 90 minutes in length. Each week there is a lesson focused primarily on one or several topics. The *Workbook* guides members through the ten-week experience, offering educational content and providing questions and space to journal responses, all of which serve as the basis for discussion during the weekly meetings.

The *Workbook* is divided into ten lessons. In a typical support group weekly meeting, one lesson is covered, although there is enough content that some of the lessons could be stretched over two or three weeks if you would prefer to cover the educational content in smaller chunks. Here is a listing of the *Workbook*'s lessons:

- Lesson One: Telling Your Story from the Beginning
- Lesson Two: Basics of Alzheimer's Disease and Other Dementias
- Lesson Three: Brain Structure and Function, Activities of Daily Living, and Dementia Stages
- Lesson Four: Adapting to Changing Relationships
- Lesson Five: Coping with Grief and Loss
- Lesson Six: Stress and Self-Care
- Lesson Seven: Getting More Help and Transitioning Care
- Lesson Eight: Legal, Financial, and End-of-Life Issues
- Lesson Nine: Existential and Spiritual Questions
- Lesson Ten: Retelling Your Story Starting Today

In our program, after completing the ten-week classroom experience, group members then may choose to transition to a counselor-led, once-a-month 90-minute "maintenance group," which is more unstructured in format. Whether you are a trained mental-health, medical, or other healthcare professional or a layperson with a heart to serve dementia care partners in either a secular or faith-based organization, as a support-group leader you can use *The Dementia Care-Partner's Workbook* and this leader's manual to help you establish a sustainable support-group program that includes the initial ten-week experience followed by monthly maintenance groups. The *Leader's Manual* provides step-by-step instructions on how to run the individual weekly meetings, general information about establishing and leading support groups, meeting-specific handouts, and lots of practical advice based on my own experiences as care partner to my late wife, Rebecca, who died in 2016 after a nine-year battle with early-onset Alzheimer's disease, as well as my career as a doctor, mental-health practitioner, and dementia care-partner support-group leader.

WHY DEMENTIA CARE-PARTNER SUPPORT GROUPS ARE IMPORTANT

A growing body of medical and mental-health research demonstrates the effectiveness of supportive-care interventions to help dementia care partners, including individual, couples, and family counseling as well as support groups. In my work at Wake Forest Baptist Health's Memory Counseling Program, I have facilitated facilitated hundreds of support gorups for dementia care partners over the last eight years and have witnessed the education, understanding, and hope exceeding members' expectations through these well-planned and well-led groups.

Support groups for dementia care partners are helpful because they:

- Introduce members to a community of others who have had similar experiences, thoughts, and feelings.
- Counter the sense of loneliness and isolation that many care partners experience.
- Provide emotional, physical, and spiritual support in a safe, nonjudgmental environment.
- Allow members to explore their many thoughts and feelings

about caregiving in ways that help them be compassionate with themselves.

- Encourage members to not only receive support and understanding for themselves but also to provide the same to others.
- Offer opportunities to learn new ways of approaching problems and challenges.
- Help them trust their fellow human beings and bond again in what for many feels like an unsafe, uncaring world.
- Give them a forum to ask questions and search for meaning.
- Provide a supportive environment that can reawaken their zest for life and give them hope for the future.

In short, as group members give and receive help, they feel less helpless themselves, are able to discover continued meaning in life, and find the energy needed to continue on their caregiving journey. Feeling understood by others brings down barriers between the dementia care partner and the outside world. This process of being understood is central to being compassionate with oneself. The more people who are compassionate to the dementia care partner from the outside in, the more they are capable of being self-compassionate from the inside out.

Support groups foster the experience of trusting and being trusted. Members can achieve a balance between giving and receiving, between independence and an appropriate, self-sustaining dependence. The group provides a safe harbor where struggling people can pull in, anchor while the wind still blows them around, and search for safe ground to manage the challenges life has brought them. As a potential leader of such a group, you have the honor of accompanying people during this time.

Before we go on to explore the specifics of running a dementia care-partner support group, I will share the framework for *The Dementia Care-Partner's Workbook*: the eight central needs of dementia care partners.

THE EIGHT CENTRAL NEEDS OF DEMENTIA CARE PARTNERS

In the introduction to *The Dementia Care-Partner's Workbook*, I describe the eight central needs of dementia care partners—eight things that my experience as care partner, counselor, and support-group leader taught me were important to each and every person who cares for a loved one with dementia. They are:

- Central Need 1—*Tell and retell your story*
- Central Need 2—*Educate yourself*
- Central Need 3—*Adapt to changing relationships*
- Central Need 4—*Grieve your losses*
- Central Need 5—*Take care of yourself*
- Central Need 6—*Ask for and accept help from others*
- Central Need 7—*Prepare for what's ahead*
- Central Need 8—*Explore existential and spiritual questions to find meaning*

Each of the ten lessons in *The Dementia Care-Partner's Workbook* focuses on one or several of the eight central needs, and by the end of the book, dementia care partners in a support group come to realize that the eight are an interwoven web of needs they have throughout their loved one's journey with dementia, some having greater relevance than others at certain points in time depending on their loved one's current symptoms and challenges. The interrelatedness of the eight central needs is the emphasis of the last lesson of the *Workbook* as well as the support group. I'll share more about this in the specific plan for Meeting Ten.

Before You Begin a Support Group

Starting a support group takes a lot of time and energy. In fact, I suspect many counselors and lay leaders alike have decided not to start a support group for dementia care partners because they didn't know where to even begin the process of establishing the group, let alone leading it.

This is precisely why I have written *The Dementia Care-Partner's Workbook* and this accompanying leader's manual. Let me share a piece of advice as you are beginning the planning process for your support group. Whether your goal is to hold a one-time, limited-duration support group or establish a sustainable, ongoing support-group program, make it a team sport by finding a committed group of people to help share the responsibilities of leading and co-leading the group and take care of the logistics needed to plan and execute it.

Here are the start-up considerations to be mindful of as you begin the planning process.

Deciding on a support-group leader

Choosing who will lead the group is the first and perhaps most important decision to make. Most often, dementia care-partner support groups are led by mental-health professionals — licensed clinical social workers or licensed professional counselors who have taken classes in group counseling during their graduate training. However, other healthcare professionals could lead the group too, such as a physician, physician assistant, nurse, nurse practitioner, or a physical, occupational, recreational, or speech therapist. Hospital or nursing-home administrators, health educators, gerontologists, geriatric case managers, or clergy could also lead. In some communities, a layperson, often someone who is or has been a dementia care partner, may want to lead.

Leading a support group takes more than the desire to do so, although that is necessary. More than their credentials, the leader should possess the necessary traits and qualities (discussed later in the *Leader's Manual*) and be willing to commit to planning for each weekly meeting. That being said, when possible, identifying someone with training and experience as group leader will give your support group the best chance of success.

It is also best to have a co-leader for the support group. Why? For several reasons. Leading a support group can be a lot of work. Having two people to plan meetings and lead the weekly activities splits the burden. If there is a problem in the group—for example, if a group member has an emotional meltdown during a meeting—the co-leader can step out with that person and give them the individual attention they need while the leader continues with the rest of the members. If the leader is sick one week, or out of town for professional reasons, instead of canceling the meeting, the co-leader could take over. It's also helpful for the leader and co-leader to debrief after meetings. The above discussion about the leader's qualifications applies to the co-leader as well. Graduate students in social work or counseling are often required to have group experience to earn their degree, and usually make excellent co-leaders. Finally, be certain that the leader and co-leader are compatible in leadership style and personality.

Needs assessment
Before making the commitment to start a dementia care-partner support group, step back and formally assess the interest for such a

group in your community. Questions to address include: What kind of support groups already exist in this community? If they do exist, they are likely to be held in residential-care settings (assisted living and memory care), adult daycare or community senior services, or through the local Alzheimer's Association, Area Agency on Aging, or PACE program. What has been the history and success of these groups? You may want to speak to the leaders of these groups to find out how well their groups have been attended, whether they used a curriculum of some sort or were more open-ended, and what worked and didn't work. Are there enough people interested in being group members? Are there individuals interested in and willing to be leaders and co-leaders?

Group format

Group format covers several different considerations, which I'll discuss in no particular order.

First, will the group be **secular or faith-based**? Most groups are secular, offered in the community to people regardless of faith orientation. Faith-based groups allow the religious practices of the particular faith community to be integrated into the group, but this may exclude members of a different faith, who might feel uncomfortable. I have noted that in African American churches, there is often a health ministry; dementia care-partner support groups are a natural extension of this.

Second, will the group **blend or separate dementia types**? As described in Lesson Two of *The Dementia Care-Partner's Workbook*, there are many different types of dementia. Alzheimer's disease is the most prevalent, followed by vascular, frontotemporal, Lewy body, and Parkinson's-disease dementia. Usually, a dementia care-partner support group will bring together care partners whose loved ones have any of these dementia types, and the *Workbook* has been written to be inclusive in this regard. However, some non-Alzheimer's care partners feel others in the group can't relate to their experience because the non-Alzheimer's dementias are so different in symptoms and challenges than Alzheimer's disease. In my experience, this perception is not necessarily true, but it is strongly held nonetheless. Hence, sometimes consideration should be given to having separate support groups for care partners of people affected by the various types of dementia. This segmentation may be feasible in a large urban area, though of course it requires more leaders and co-leaders.

Third, will the group be **psychoeducational**? Support groups based on *The Dementia Care-Partner's Workbook* are psychoeducational groups. Psychoeducational groups are made up of like-individuals (in this case, dementia care partners) and focus on providing education and understanding about a particular topic (dementia), with the goal of enhancing coping skills by processing members' thoughts and emotions. There are also other types of support groups, such as self-help, therapy, and social support groups, that may be appropriate for dementia care partners as well, but a discussion of them is beyond the scope of *A Leader's Manual*.

Last, will the group be **open or closed**? There are two types of support group structures: "open," meaning that the group is open to whomever wishes to come (and go) on a week-to-week basis depending on their needs, and "closed," meaning a set number of members are enrolled, typically for a defined period of time, and the group is closed to others once it has begun. As I described previously, the dementia care-partner support group program at Wake Forest Baptist Health involves an initial ten-week classroom experience, which is a closed group, followed by monthly maintenance support groups, which are open. My bias is that the closed structure works best and is the premise for the ten lessons that make up *The Dementia Care-Partner's Workbook*. Members in closed groups feel the most comfortable, and the group is more likely to develop a sense of intimacy, both of which translate into the best possible group experience. The open structure works well in maintenance groups, even when members have come from different ten-week groups. I'll discuss maintenance groups more in a later section of *A Leader's Manual*.

Choosing a place and time of day to meet

Finding a comfortable, safe place to hold group meetings is probably the second most important decision to be made. Public buildings such as libraries, schools, and community centers usually provide rooms free-of-charge. Faith communities such as churches, synagogues, mosques, and temples are also willing to provide free space. Ease of parking and handicapped accessibility are important considerations for dementia care-partner support groups, since some members will be older and may have mobility challenges.

Try to select a room appropriate for creating a supportive atmosphere, neither too large nor too small and preferably distraction-free, away from heavy traffic areas. Also, pay attention to both the height of the ceiling and the lighting. Very high ceilings and bright overhead lights often make for a lack of warmth and intimacy. A large whiteboard may be handy, especially if the group leader's style is to highlight or supplement what's in each lesson's text. A computer projector and sound system for the room might also be a consideration if the group leader decides to integrate content from the internet, YouTube, DVDs, PowerPoint slides, or the like.

The time of day meetings are held is also an important consideration. For care partners who are older and retired, mid-to-late morning or early-to-mid afternoon usually works best. In contrast, adult children who are care partners typically prefer late-afternoon or early-evening meetings. You may want to include a question about the best time of day to meet when doing your needs assessment.

Setting the number of members

The number of support group members will be related to the kind and quality of interaction that is desired. When groups are too small, especially if members are not talkative, there may not be the critical mass needed to have discussion and sharing of thoughts, feelings, and ideas. When groups get too large, the sense of safety and freedom to be verbally expressive diminishes for many people. In addition, I feel it is very important for every group member to have the opportunity to speak every time the group meets; large groups preclude this. All this being said, the optimum group size in my experience is eight to 16 people, or 12 on average. If the dementia care-partner support group is new to your organization or community, and/or if you have inexperienced leaders/co-leaders, keep the first group to no more than 12 members, ideally eight to ten, before trying to tackle a larger group.

Deciding on the number of lessons and frequency and length of meetings

The Dementia Care-Partner's Workbook, as written, provides ten weekly lessons. I have experimented with groups that have had as few as four to six weekly meetings, and as many as 12, and have found that ten weekly meetings works best. That being said, the curriculum is flexible. The leader could omit certain lessons at their choosing for a shorter group, though I would not recommend fewer than four to six meetings. In contrast, there is enough content in each lesson that a group could easily extend beyond ten meetings.

My experience also has taught me that each meeting should run somewhere between 90 minutes and two hours. Assuming the member's loved one with dementia is at home with another family member, a friend, or a paid caregiver, the member will be pressed for time and will prefer the 90-minute meeting length (unless there is a provision for on-site care for the person with dementia). Obviously, larger groups require more time so that every member has a chance to talk.

Most groups meet weekly, but other frequencies, such as biweekly or monthly, are also possible. Once again, experience has taught me that the ten weekly meetings corresponding to the ten lessons in *The Dementia Care-Partner's Workbook* provide the best group and individual experiences. Biweekly or monthly meetings often result in a high attrition rate because the infrequency can't foster that essential sense of routine, comfort, and commitment. On the other hand, the maintenance groups work extremely well meeting just once a month.

Recruiting and screening group members

Not every dementia care partner makes a good support-group member. Some may be in shock or even denial about their loved one's diagnosis. Some are struggling with substance use or abuse, or have serious mental-health challenges of their own. They are best helped by individual counseling. Who is admitted to the group is a judgment call, and sometimes, despite best intentions, a member may be allowed into the group who has to be asked to leave to pursue individual counseling.

On way to avoid problematic group members is to prescreen them, which we routinely do in the Memory Counseling Program for all of our support groups. A quick ten-to-15-minute telephone screen usually suffices. This is a great job for the co-leader to do! This allows the screener to tell the potential member about the group and what it entails, stress the importance of attending all meetings, ask about emotional challenges (are they experiencing severe depression, anxiety, and/or stress that would prevent them from participating in the group), and state one of the group's ground rules—that members must attend "clean and sober." Prescreening has the added benefit of making members who attend the group at ease, because they already know one of the leaders when they come to the initial meeting.

Alternatively, the screening can be done following the first group meeting. It is usually apparent when a member is not well-suited for the group. They can be spoken with privately after the first meeting, gently told why now may not be the best time for them to be in the group, and set up for individual counseling, with the hope that they can participate in a future group. However, with this approach, you risk alienating the other group members, particularly if the member who had to be excused was highly emotional or confrontational during the first meeting.

Strategies to publicize the group

There are a number of strategies you can use to publicize a support group, many of which are free, though others can be quite expensive. Try any or all of the following:

- Word-of-mouth
  This is often how many if not most of your potential members will learn about the group—they hear from another dementia care partner who is in an ongoing group and sings its praises!

- Direct communication with medical/mental-health professionals and clergy
  Start by identifying the professionals in your community who work with dementia patients and their care partners. Let them and their clinical and office staff know about your support group.

  Dementia is usually diagnosed by a neurologist, psychiatrist, geriatrician, or neuropsychologist, although many primary-care doctors, such as family practitioners or internists, make dementia diagnoses as well. Inquiry into the local medical community can usually determine who the main dementia doctors are.

  Another professional group to target for referral to your group are mental-health professionals, including licensed clinical social workers, licensed professional counselors, and psychologists, whose practices include or are focused on geriatric clients, including those with dementia. Once again, inquiring into the mental-health community can usually identify who these individuals are. Clergy can be similarly targeted with this approach.

  In addition to speaking personally with all of these professionals and/ or their staff (a brief face-to-face or phone conversation will suffice), they may allow you to place posters, flyers, and/or brochures about your support group in their offices.

- Local media
  Most communities have a newspaper that provides a community calendar that will announce the group, provide a brief description about it, and explain how to contact the leader or co-leader responsible for additional information and prescreening. Or, you can purchase space on a page to advertise the group, although this can be

very expensive. The newspaper editor may even be willing to feature a short article about the group, especially if it is a new group in the community.

Radio and TV stations may also have the equivalent of a community calendar or a way to buy air time to feature the group. If your organization has a media specialist, a press release could be written and sent to local newspapers, radio, and TV stations.

- **Posters, flyers, and brochures**
Posters, flyers, and brochures are other effective ways of marketing a dementia care-partner support group. Logical places to post them include residential-care facilities, such as assisted living and memory care, nursing homes, senior-living and continuing-care retirement communities, adult daycare centers, places of worship, and any other location unique to your area where there is a high concentration of older adults or people with dementia.

- **The internet**
Last, but certainly not least, is the internet. If you are a community agency sponsoring the dementia care-partner support group and have your own website, create a unique link to a full-page description of the support group. If possible, provide a phone number or email address so interested community members can contact the group leader, co-leader, or an administrative contact, or provide a form for people to type in their contact information so someone can reach out to them. This may require the assistance of a webmaster. The webmaster or another expert in websites can also help with search-engine optimization, the process by which individuals in your area who search "dementia support groups" or something similar on the internet will be directed to your agency's website.

You might also want to compile a group email list comprised of area healthcare professionals as well as dementia care partners. With one click you will be able to disseminate group information, including an attached flyer .pdf and contact information.

Use of the internet and email to reach potential support group members is the least personal but most efficient way to disseminate group information and recruit members.

Establishing ground rules

By prescreening members and having a set of ground rules for the group to abide by, you can create a safe and ideal setting for the support-group experience. Ground rules are also important tools for group leaders. For example, should someone begin to verbally dominate the group, the leader can remind the talkative member of the ground rules that ensure all members will have equal time to express themselves. Ground rules should be discussed early in the very first meeting. As a reminder, they can even be posted in the room where group is held. Sample ground rules are provided in Appendix 1. Feel free to use or modify them depending on the needs and wants of your group leader and members.

Baseline and end-of-group assessments

While I feel confident that most members who complete *The Dementia Care-Partner's Workbook* ten-week support-group experience will find it immensely beneficial, you may want to measure this by using baseline and end-of-group assessments. There are two kinds of assessments you can use: those measuring member characteristics—such as levels of burden, depression, and anxiety before and after the group—and others that evaluate the member's experience with the support group, curriculum, and leaders.

Below are descriptions of the core assessment instruments we use at Wake Forest Baptist Health in our Memory Counseling Program dementia care-partner support groups. They are provided in Appendices 2 and 3 of *A Leader's Manual*. Each form takes several up to ten minutes to complete. One option is to have members fill them out during the first and last meetings, which results in the best compliance but takes up valuable group time. Alternatively, you could hand them out during the first and last meetings and ask that they be returned in preaddressed envelopes you provide (however, about a third of group members won't complete or return them).

Here are some additional suggestions if more robust research instruments are desired: depression (Patient Health Questionnaire [PHQ]-9 and Beck Depression Inventory), anxiety (Generalized Anxiety Disorder [GAD]-7 and Beck Anxiety Inventory), stress (Perceived Stress Scale), and grief (Marwit-Meuser Caregiver Grief Index Short Form).

- Zarit Caregiver Burden Scale (Appendix 2)—This is the most widely used instrument to measure care-partner burden. It has 22 questions—for example, "Do you feel stressed between caring for your relative and trying to meet other responsibilities for your family or work?"—with individual responses scaled from 0 to 4 resulting in a total score of 0 to 88. Total scores are interpreted as follows: 0-20, no/little burden; 21-40, mild-moderate burden; 41-60, moderate-severe burden; and 61-88, severe burden.

- Geriatric Depression Scale (GDS) and Geriatric Anxiety Scale (GAS) (Appendix 3) —These are commonly used screening tools to assess depressive and anxious symptoms in older adults. Each has 15 questions with yes or no responses, so the total score ranges from 0 to 15. For the GDS, score 1 point for a "yes" response to questions 2-4, 6, 8-10, 12, 14, and 15, and "no" responses to questions 1, 5, 7, 11, and 13. For the GAS, score 1 point for a "yes" response to questions 1-4, 6, 8-10, 12, 14, and 15, and "no" responses to questions 5, 7, 11, and 13. Total scores are interpreted as follows: a score of 5 or above on either scale indicates the presence of mild-moderate (total score 5-10) to severe (11-15) depressive/anxious symptoms.

If you use the Zarit Caregiver Burden and Geriatric Depression/Anxiety Scales, scores for individuals in the group as well as the group as a whole can be compared at baseline versus end-of-group.

Basic Skills of the Support-Group Leader

In the prior section, we covered the myriad tasks that need to be done in order to establish a dementia care-partner support group. The importance of choosing a support-group leader was discussed. Now let's turn our attention to the leader him- or herself—their responsibilities, qualities, style, and skills they will use to lead. We'll also talk about the important notion of *companioning*.

Responsibilities of the support-group leader

The overarching responsibility of the support-group leader is to create a safe and ideal setting for care partners to connect, share, learn, become resilient, and gather strength to continue on the journey companioning their loved one with dementia. Sensitive, skilled leadership is vital to the group's success. Specific leader responsibilities, which can be shared between the leader and co-leader, include the following (keeping in mind that every group has its own unique requirements):

- Set the tone for the group. Members will sense the interest, desire, effort, and passion of the group leader. They will perceive the leader's "way of being" and follow their lead.

- Plan and lead group meetings. The leader will help determine the group's purpose and length, prescreen members, and develop ground rules as well as prepare for, organize, and facilitate the group meetings.

- Understand and facilitate group process. The group leader must possess both the attributes and skills of a capable group leader. They must have some content expertise, a basic knowledge of aging and dementia, as well as a basic knowledge of group process. A group leader committed to organizing and running a sustainable support-group program participates in lifelong training opportunities to hone existing skills and develop new ones.

- Model good listening skills, openness, and caring. The leader must really hear what members are saying, consciously opening themselves up to being taught what members are thinking and feeling on the inside and encouraging them to express themselves freely by being heard in a warm, caring, and empathetic manner.

- Respond to conflicts and problems that arise in the group, and sense when the group is not making progress or is "stuck." The leader must guide the group through difficulties that arise, responding appropriately to damaging behavior that may occur in the group and/or modifying or adapting meeting plans when the group is not making progress.

- Follow up with members outside of the group. Some group members may need extra time, which can happen informally before or after weekly group meetings, whereas others may need referral for individual counseling either during the course of the support group or after it has ended.

If you are an organization and have committed to starting a dementia care-partner support group program but have not yet selected a leader, let me re-emphasize how important it is to find the right person for this position. If necessary, create a job description (the responsibilities outlined above can help you model the document) and use it to recruit the best person possible. Effective leaders find the opportunity to shepherd a group through the ten weeks of *The Dementia Care-Partner's Workbook* curriculum and make it a meaningful and enjoyable experience.

Qualities of the support-group leader

One of the foundational qualities an effective support-group leader must have is the ability to communicate well. To be helpful to your group members, a leader must communicate with them effectively and make them feel both cared for and about.

We all have observed people whom we would call "natural helpers." Actually, the helping skills that seem so natural to them are more likely the personality traits they were born with or habits they've learned and developed over time. The most important helping quality is empathy, but there are others described below, as well. Almost anyone with a teachable spirit and the willingness to learn can develop the helping qualities they need to be an effective support-group leader.

- **Empathy**

  Empathy is the ability to perceive another's experience and then—this is the key—communicate that perception back to the person. As a support-group leader, I listen to members, and though I cannot directly experience what they experience, I begin to have a mental picture of the essence of what they are describing by imagining it from their perspective—that is, through their eyes, not mine.

  Perhaps the most vital part of this characteristic is the ability to convey accurate empathy. Empathetic responsiveness requires the ability to go beyond factual detail and to become involved in the other person's feeling world, but always with the "as if" quality of taking on another's role without personally experiencing what the other person experiences (if you actually experienced the same emotions as the person you are trying to help, you would be overinvolved). To have empathy for another person does not constitute the direct expression of one's own feelings, but rather focuses exclusively on the feelings expressed by another. In other words, conveying an empathetic understanding of them.

  Good leaders know that empathy has been communicated when group members feel that the leader "understands" them. As you know, to say simply "I understand how you feel" is not enough. Members must perceive at a gut emotional level that to some degree, the leader is feeling and thinking as they are, which is communicated both verbally and nonverbally. We'll talk more about specific verbal and nonverbal skills a bit later in *A Leader's Manual.*

- Respectfulness
  Respect is the ability to communicate the belief that everyone has inherent value as well as both the capacity and right to choose and make their own decisions. Respect requires a non-possessive caring for and affirmation of another person. It means respecting another's right to be who and what they are, even if they are very different than you. This quality involves a receptive attitude that embraces the other person's thoughts, feelings, opinions, and uniqueness—even those radically different from yours.

  So, the dimension of respect is communicated when support-group members feel they have been allowed to give input without being pressured and when their opinions have been considered important. Remembering what the person has said, demonstrating sensitivity and courtesy, and showing respect for the person's feelings and beliefs are the essences of communicating respect.

- Warmth and caring
  The warm and caring support-group leader cultivates a sense of personal closeness, as opposed to professional distance, with group members. Showing warmth and caring is particularly helpful in the early phases of building a helping relationship with group members. The dimension of warmth is communicated primarily nonverbally. It often has to do with affect, facial expression, posture, and other nonverbal cues.

  Warmth is a very powerful dimension in the helping process. In fact, when a discrepancy exists between verbal and nonverbal behavior, people almost always believe the nonverbal (this is also true of people who have dementia—they will almost always focus more on what they see than what they hear). A person's nonverbal behavior seldom lies. Consequently, a person who has excellent verbal communication skills but lacks "warm" nonverbal behavior would more than likely be perceived by group members as not helpful, indifferent, cold, or uncaring.

- **Genuineness**

  Genuineness is the ability to present oneself sincerely. As a support-group leader, this is your ability to be freely yourself—without phoniness, role playing, or defensiveness. It's when your outer words and behaviors match your inner feelings.

  The dimension of genuineness involves disclosing how you feel about an issue. One important caveat: try not to tell others how you feel too early because your opinion may interfere with their ability to open up and express their own unique and equally valid thoughts and feelings. Genuineness can be very helpful, but timing is important. You can earn the right to be genuine with others through first developing your relationship with them.

- **Trustworthiness**

  In addition to the qualities described thus far in this section, a responsible and effective support-group leader also needs to create conditions for mutual trust to naturally develop and grow not only between leaders and members, but also within the group among members. One important way is by facilitating the honoring of stories (remember Central Need 1 of dementia care partners is the need to tell and retell their story, and it's the main focus of Lessons One and Ten of *The Dementia Care-Partner's Workbook*). It is through the personal experiences of the members that people do the "work" of a group, a concept that will be described in much greater detail in the subsequent section of *A Leader's Manual* on the stages or phases of a support group. The more time the group is given to share their stories, the deeper the expression of feelings will be, and the more rapidly the group's trust, relationships, and sense of community will grow.

Naturally, as trust builds, members feel more comfortable expressing a multitude of thoughts and feelings, although effective leadership means recognizing that personal sharing may be difficult for some, so members are never forced to participate but rather are encouraged and supported when doing so. In the beginning, members tend to express "safer" feelings, but as trust increases, they are willing to be more vulnerable and share feelings such as fear, helplessness, and anger. Obviously, as members take greater risks in expressing themselves and continue to experience compassion and empathy from other members as well as the group leader, community grows.

A support-group leader can create an atmosphere for authentic emotional expression by praising support-group members when they respond compassionately to one another and encouraging other members to do the same. As the group members witness the support in action from the leaders as well as fellow members, they will come to realize that the group is a place in which they can honestly express whatever trials and tribulations they are facing as dementia care partners.

Model for members that it is not their responsibility to solve each other's problems but instead to support one another as they encounter the challenges of dementia caregiving. When members realize they can share their own struggles or bear witness to the struggles of others without others receiving or giving unsolicited advice, they are more likely to trust each other and the group process.

And finally, to maintain trust, don't hesitate to revisit group ground rules when necessary. This is particularly true when it comes to confidentiality, perhaps the most important rule of all. Sound leadership requires that members understand how important it is not to repeat to others what group members express in the group. Model confidentiality, (re)emphasize its importance, and remind members that without confidentiality, there will be no trust.

Defining leadership style

The personality of support-group leaders and co-leaders can vary widely, from gregarious and **extroverted**, taking a very visible role in leading the group, to more passive and **introverted**, preferring more to blend in with other group members. Which is best? In truth, probably somewhere in between.

A leader who talks so much that members don't have the opportunity to share is as ineffective as one who says so little that members aren't sure what they're supposed to do. The most effective leaders let members know that someone is in charge. They are firm and provide direction without being obtrusive, yet are warm and caring, genuine, and empathetically responsive. Their focus is always on the health of the group—that is, that making sure the group is a safe and ideal setting for care partners to connect, share, learn, become resilient, and gather strength to continue on the journey caring for their loved one with dementia.

Two other important qualities of an effective group leader are **flexibility and the ability to share authority**. Being flexible is important because some meetings—no matter how much advance preparation is done—will not go as planned because of how individuals in the group or the group as a whole responds during discussion. Sometimes the group may go in a different direction than anticipated, especially for well-established groups where members have developed enough intimacy to share very openly. A good leader never rigidly places their own agenda for the group ahead of needs that the group develops organically.

The ability and willingness of the group leader to share their role is also very important. We've already discussed the importance of a co-leader. In addition, sometimes one or two members of a group will want to take a more active role, as unofficial co-leaders. This must be done very thoughtfully or it can undermine the group and its normal development. Seeking the opinion of a particularly wise or thoughtful group member is a good way to initiate or augment a discussion, and having group members question one another and freely share between themselves should always be encouraged. But having a member function as an unofficial co-leader might make other members feel left out or perceive favoritism has occurred. Sharing leadership responsibilities, like being flexible, is a quality of a good leader who puts the health of the group first and intervenes and redirects if the group dynamic becomes unhealthy.

Basic counseling skills of the support-group leader

In addition to the innate and learned support-group leader qualities already described, there are a number of skills that support-group leaders need to learn and practice in order to be the most effective they can be. Skills can be used to "make something happen," or they can be used to elaborate on what is already happening. In other words, *skills are a means, not an end.*

If you are a trained mental-health professional, you have most likely had a class on group counseling and both learned and practiced these skills in a supervised setting. For lay support-group leaders, learning these skills is a bit more challenging. Ideally, in your first support-group experience you'd be a co-leader working with an experienced support-group leader who can take the time to teach you these skills, model them for you, and discuss them with you after you've observed their use in the group setting.

You can also attend a support-group leader training offered by the Center for Loss and Life Transition with Dr. Wolfelt (www.centerforloss. com/trainings). Although the training has a grief focus, it is fully applicable to dementia care-partner support groups and by 2020, I plan to be offering a support-group leader training course based on *The Dementia Care-Partner's Workbook* and *A Leader's Manual.* For information on my course as it evolves, visit empatheducation.com.

OK, let's jump into the skills themselves. The following is a summary of the most important skills for a support-group leader to know and use, adapted with permission from Dr. Samuel Gladding's book on groups listed in the Resources section. If you want to dig deeper, I would suggest reading further in Gladding's book as well as the other resources noted.

For each of the skills listed below, you will be given the name of the skill, a description of it, its aim or desired outcome, and an example of how the skill can be used. Here we go!

- **Active listening** is the skill of attending to verbal and nonverbal aspects of communication without judging or evaluating. Its aim is to encourage trust and member self-disclosure and exploration. For example: "Bill, I hear what you're saying, and I can see that you're experiencing some tears. Can you tell me what your tears are for?" As an aside, whenever you encounter a group member crying, don't assume what their tears are for—rather, ask them.

- **Restating** is the skill of saying in slightly different words what a member has said in order to clarify its meaning. The aim is to determine whether the leader has understood the member's statement correctly, and to provide support and clarification. "Mary, so your sister's main symptoms thus far have been short-term memory loss, difficulty multitasking, and some wayfinding problems while driving? I want to be sure I heard you correctly."

- **Clarifying** is the skill of grasping the essence of a message at both the thinking and feeling levels, and simplifying the member's statements by focusing on the core of their message. The aim is to help members sort out conflicting and confused thoughts and feelings, and to arrive at a meaningful understanding of what is being communicated. For example: "William, when your wife no longer knew you as her husband and you had to sleep in separate beds, you felt the intimacy in your relationship was gone?"

- **Summarizing and paraphrasing** are skills that pull together the important elements described by an individual member or the group as a whole. The aim is to avoid fragmentation and give direction to a meeting, as well as to provide for continuity and meaning. For example: "So group, a number of you have given examples of how lonely and isolated you feel as dementia care partners. This is a common experience, though an uncomfortable one."

- **Questioning** is a skill in which open-ended questions are asked that lead to self-exploration of the "what" and "how" of behavior. For example: "Susan, how did you feel the first time you had to change your mom's soiled pull-up?"

- **Interpreting** is a skill that offers possible explanations for certain thoughts, feelings, and things others say and do. The aim is to encourage deeper self-exploration, and to provide a new perspective for considering and understanding someone's behavior. For example: "John, given the stage of your wife's dementia, perhaps she hit you out of frustration rather than anger or hatred. What do you think?"

- **Confronting and reality testing** is a skill in which members are challenged to look at discrepancies between their words and actions, or verbal communication and body language. The aim is to make members aware of contradictions and encourage honest introspection. For example: "Betty, I hear you say that you've accepted Bob's dementia diagnosis, but you look very upset. Maybe you could tell me more about what you're thinking and feeling right now."

- **Reflecting feelings** is a skill in which the leader communicates understanding of the content of the member's feelings. The aim is to let the member know that they are heard and understood beyond what the leader's words can convey. For example: "Cynthia, you've shared that your mom, her mom, and your maternal great-grandmother all had Alzheimer's disease. This must be so frightening for you."

- **Supporting** is a skill in which encouragement and reinforcement are provided to the member. The aim is to create an atmosphere that will encourage the member to continue desired behaviors, provide help when they are facing difficult struggles, and encourage trust.

For example: "Jill, you have become much more effective responding to your dad's paranoia about you stealing money from him with the acknowledge-affirm-redirect strategy. Keep up the good work!"

- **Empathizing** is a skill we've already discussed, but to summarize, it's when the leader identifies with members by assuming their frames of reference. The aim is to foster trust between leader and member, communicate understanding, and encourage deeper levels of self-exploration. For example: "Ben, I can see and hear how you're struggling to care for your dad's basic needs and help him maintain his dignity. I'm sorry. Let's talk about the kinds of help that may be available to lighten your load as you help your father with his toileting and showering."

- **Facilitating, linking, and initiating** are three related skills that enhance communication in the group by increasing interaction among members and helping them assume more responsibility for the group's direction. The aim is to promote communication among group members, increase the pace of group process, and help members reach their goals for participating in the group. For example: "Samantha, now that you've shared with the group strategies for dealing with your mom's sundowning, perhaps you could ask Kim and Bill what their approach has been to their parents' sundowning and then summarize for the group."

- **Goal-setting** is a skill in which plans are made for specific goals, either for individual members or the group as a whole. The aim is to give direction to individuals and the group. For example: "I'd like each of you to find one situation between now and next week's meeting to practice being patient with your loved one. We'll discuss your examples next week during check-in."

- **Evaluating and giving feedback** are skills in which the group's accomplishments (or lack thereof) and dynamics are assessed by the group leader with the aim of promoting deeper self-awareness for individuals in the group and the group as a whole. For example: "I'm sensing that most of you are struggling with too much to do and not enough time to do it. I can sense the frustration and fatigue you are feeling, both of which are common for the care partners of loved ones with early-onset dementia. Let's take the rest of today's meeting to talk about ways you've been successful in managing your time while also meeting your family's needs and taking some time for self-care."

- **Suggesting** is a skill in which the leader offers advice, information, direction, and ideas for new behavior. It helps members develop alternative ways of thinking and responding to specific situations. For example: "Maranda, maybe you could try offering your sister just two menu choices when you take her out to a restaurant. At her stage of dementia, it's hard for her to read and remember so many different options of what to eat."

- **Protecting and blocking** are related skills in which the leader safeguards members from unwanted or counterproductive behaviors that may occur in the group. The aim is to reduce the likelihood of, or prevent unnecessary harmful psychological risks to group members. For example: "Al, we respect your choice to give Emily coconut oil, but remember we caution against advice giving in our group ground rules. Suggesting that everyone in the group should give their loved one two tablespoons of coconut oil daily may be an unhealthy recommendation."

- **Self-disclosure** is a skill in which the leader shares personal information, such as their experiences or views, to the group. The aim is to provide information that the leader feels will be helpful to members in some way—for example, modeling a certain behavior. It should not be used as a way for the leader to share information about themselves for their own benefit or to join the group as a member (this can be particularly challenging for lay support-group leaders or co-leaders). An example of healthy self-disclosure is the following: "It sounds as though several of you are battling depression. From personal experience, I'm aware of how challenging some of the symptoms can be."

- **Modeling** is a skill in which a desired behavior is demonstrated through action. The aim is to provide examples of helpful behavior and, depending on what's being modeled, to inspire members to fully develop their potential. Here's an example of modeling that includes self-disclosure too: "I've found mindfulness to be a helpful way to cope with my depression. By taking a Mindfulness Moment each morning and evening, when getting up and right when I go to bed, I feel much more grounded. Let me demonstrate my mindfulness routine to you."

- **Silence** is a skill in which the leader refrains from both verbal and nonverbal reflection. The aim is to allow group members to process emotionally intense content or experiences, reflect, and tap into the strength of the group as a whole. For example: "Wow, what Casey and Brad shared was both thought-provoking and challenging. Let's take a couple of moments to silently think about what they've said before we process it as a group."

- **Terminating** is the skill used to prepare the group for the last meeting in which they will meet together. The aim is to prepare group members to transition back to pre-group life, hopefully with a new set of coping skills, feeling safe and secure. For example: "Today is the last of our ten meetings. Let's take a few minutes to talk about what the group has meant to you, as well as any apprehensions you may have about navigating your caregiving journey without the support the group has provided you these last few months."

You may feel overwhelmed by all of these skills. The differences between some of them may seem unclear or subtle. In reality, when you are leading a support group, using these skills often comes quite naturally, especially after some real-life experience in the field.

The nature and art of companioning

The model of care used in *The Dementia Care-Partner's Workbook* and *A Leader's Manual* is a soulful, holistic approach called "companioning," originally developed by Dr. Wolfelt as a model of bereavement care for those who have experienced grief and loss through the death of a loved one.

The companioning model of care can also be applied to counseling dementia care partners, whether it be on an individual level or in the setting of a support group. As Dr. Wolfelt explains, companioning is about:

- Honoring the spirit, not focusing on intellect.
- Curiosity, not expertise.
- Learning from others, not teaching them.
- Walking alongside, not leading.
- Being still, not frantically moving forward.
- Discovering the gifts of sacred silence, not filling every painful moment with words.
- Listening with the heart, not analyzing with the head.
- Bearing witness to the struggles of others, not directing those struggles.
- Being present to another person's struggles and pain, not taking them away.
- Respecting disorder and confusion, not order and logic.
- Turning inward and going into the wilderness of the soul with another human being, not thinking you are responsible for helping them find the way out.

If you as support-group leader companion the dementia care partner, you allow them to experience their burden, depression, anxiety, stress, grief, and loss of control, while searching for meaning and finding the strength to keep on keeping on—which, on a given day, may only be overcoming the inertia to get their feet out of bed. I encourage you to embrace the companioning philosophy in your heart and make it the foundation on which you lead.

Support Group
Basics

In the prior section, we focused on the support-group leader. In this section, we'll focus on the support group itself, including topics such as the basic needs of support-group members, the developmental phases or stages of a support group, and challenges that are encountered when leading a support group. Let's begin.

Basic needs of support-group members

In the Introduction section, we talked about why dementia care-partner support groups are important. The support-group leader's job is to create a safe and ideal setting for care partners to connect, share, learn, become resilient, and gather strength to continue on the journey caring for their loved one with dementia.

To accomplish this, the members' basic needs must be met. What are the basic needs of support group members that must be addressed for the group to be successful? They are:

- Each member must understand the purpose of the group.

- Each member must feel a sense of belonging and acceptance.

- Each member must feel understood and valued.

- Each member must be aware of and respectful of the ground rules, especially the importance of confidentiality ("what's said in the group stays in the group").

- Each member must feel encouraged to be an active member in the group (while respecting "quiet" members).

- Each member must be able to see the faces of all the other members (so arrange the seating appropriately).

I'm sure you can think of other basic needs too, but these are the essential ones. Now let's talk about a support group's developmental phases.

The five developmental phases of a support group

Why is it important to understand that support groups go through developmental phases? Because knowledge of these phases allows you to both respect and nurture the natural unfolding of the group's development. For example, if you were to expect in-depth self-exploration of all members at the first meeting, you would not be respecting the reality that this kind of sharing generally does not happen until group trust has been established over time.

Although the developmental phases typically occur sequentially, there is also a cyclical aspect of the group's evolution. For example, dementia care-partners' Central Need 1—Tell and retell their story—is important in each of the curriculum's ten weekly meetings. As members share their stories in successive meetings, they emphasize different aspects, with progressively deeper levels of meaning, each time.

With this background, let's review the five developmental phases of a group, presented in the context of a dementia care-partners support group.

- PHASE ONE (forming):
  Warm-up and establishing group purpose and limits
  When a support group is forming, it is normal for members to feel anxious and have some uncertainty about what is to come. "What will happen here? What is the purpose?" they wonder. Group members may be questioning their capacity to hear about or take on the burdens of others, let alone their own. Be aware that some group members

will attend with a certain amount of hesitancy or resistance and may question whether or not they should even be there.

Among the other questions that may go through their minds during this phase are, "Who else is in this group? Will I know them? How does their care-partnering experience compare to mine? Will they understand me or judge me? Will I feel comfortable with these people? What will we talk about? What can and can't be said? Are there certain expectations the group will have of me? Will the leader make it 'safe' for me to just be who I am? Will I have to talk, even if at times I don't want to? Can I trust the people in this group?" As the answers to these questions become clear, members begin to feel they understand the nature and limits of the group.

Behaviorally, members will tend to reflect their unique personalities. Some will be more expressive, while others may be silent and withdrawn. This initial period of getting to know each other is critical for what will or will not follow. By promoting positive interactions among members, you will be helping members actively participate in each meeting and continue coming to subsequent meetings.

The leader plays a critical role in making it safe during this initial phase of the group's development. Here the primary leadership roles include:

- Clarifying the purpose of the group.
- Being aware of members' anxiety and apprehension.
- Asking what each group member's expectations and goals are for their group experience.
- Gently encouraging each member to tell their story.
- Creating the ground rules for the group, and sharing the rules with group members, emphasizing confidentiality.
- Modeling listening and helping everyone feel as if they belong.
- Facilitating details such as the time the meetings will begin, how

long they will be, what the general format of each meeting is, and the like.

- PHASE TWO (storming):
Tentative self-disclosure and exploring group boundaries
This is the phase where members begin to learn what is expected to happen in the group. Every group has expectations (spoken and unspoken) about what will happen in the group meeting. Essentially, members are learning how to be *participating* members of the support group.

During this phase members begin to see themselves as a group and disclose more about themselves and their journeys as dementia care partners. Often this self-disclosure is rather tentative. Members are exploring the boundaries of whether it's safe or risky to be more vulnerable when moving to a deeper level of self-disclosure.

This phase of self-disclosure and exploring group boundaries is also called the storming stage because conflict may arise between group members. Not all groups experience storming, but if they do, that week or two can be the most challenging for the leaders. Differences in members' personalities, their communication styles, and healthy and unhealthy ways of coping become more apparent now that they've moved beyond the initial forming stage. Conflict may arise between the leader and members as well as between members themselves. Certain personality types among members tend to promote conflict, such Ann the Advice-Giver, Albert the Academic, and Ivan the Interrupter, or lead to resistance engaging in the group, like Molly the Missing or Fred the Forced. We'll talk more about these and other challenging individuals and their personalities a bit later in this section.

Through increasing self-disclosure and the exploring of group boundaries, members begin to learn more about each other, the leader, and themselves.

During this phase the primary leadership roles include:

- Continuing to clarify member goals and expectations of the group.
- Reminding members of the ground rules established at the first meeting.
- Continuing to model listening, openness, and caring, especially when encountering anxious or apprehensive members.
- Being responsive to conflicts, resistance, or other problems that might arise.

- PHASE THREE (norming):
  In-depth self-exploration and confronting the realities of caregiving.
  As the group grows and develops, a subtle but important movement takes place. The group begins to move away from the initial discovery of the "why" of the group, past the exploration of boundaries and conflicts. It is during this time that in-depth self-exploration occurs, and the raw emotion associated with the challenges of being a care partner to someone with a progressive, ultimately fatal neurodegenerative disease emerges. In this phase, interactions between members typically become more intense and emotional. A higher rate of interpersonal self-disclosure and in-depth self-expression is now taking place. Members are vulnerable but trusting when they share. The group shifts into high gear, evolving group trust at a deeper level.

During this phase, a natural insider/outsider feeling often begins to develop, and certain members may begin to express how important the group is to them. Now the group is feeling good about itself, and members look forward to each meeting. Being part of a group with other dementia care partners feels good and normal (hence the norming stage). At this point members are much more likely to ask questions of and speak directly to one another, bypassing the leader as they collaborate with their co-journeyers on how to handle a particular challenge or cope in healthier ways. Cohesion among members and the group as a whole is developing. Unofficial co-leaders within the group may even begin to emerge. This too is normal, though an inexperienced or unconfident leader may feel threatened by this.

At this point, you as leader may have to become more supportively confrontive with problem members who try to detour the group from its primary purposes.

With any luck this phase of the group will last for weeks. When the group reaches and is in this norming stage, leaders can breathe a sigh of relief; it's where they hope every group will land after the forming and storming have occurred.

Leadership roles during this phase include:

- Continuing to model listening, openness, and caring.
- Being supportive of continued participation of group members.
- Being responsive to conflicts, resistance, or other problems that might arise (some storming can still occur during the norming stage).
- Encouraging communication between group members by using the skills of facilitating, linking, and initiating (refer back to the basic skills section).
- Allowing and encouraging the group to be more self-responsible.
- Making appropriate adjustments to content and format based on the direction the group wants to go or is taking itself.

- PHASE FOUR (working):
  Commitment to healing and growth
  Whereas in the prior phase members' exploration is often in-depth, allowing them to experience the deep pain, emotion, and grief of being a dementia care partner, in this next phase, another subtle but important movement takes place—toward healing and growth. During this phase, which occurs during the last few meetings, just

prior to the group's end, interaction among group members is at its peak. Many members begin to ask for and reach out to others for mutual help and support. There is a sense of trust and togetherness. Members have discovered that they are resilient and can survive the challenges of being a care partner to their spouse or parent with dementia. They even realize that with some changes in what they think, say, and do, they can integrate self-care and wellness back into their lives as they strive for more balance. The group ambiance takes on a more relaxed tone. Members feel safe and "at home" in the group. If conflict arises, they are able to address it in healthy ways.

Phase Four is clearly the most valuable phase in the life of the dementia care-partner support group. The group is working in several senses. Earlier concerns and developmental phases have been achieved, and the group is moving at a faster pace. Respect and trust levels are way up, which allows members to share what they need to share with much more honest and open "I" expressions of thoughts and feelings about their successes and failures as care partners. They gain insights as individuals but share them with the group, and in doing so, crystallize the group's cohesion.

By this time members are genuinely concerned about the well-being of other members. Group members will also often express their feelings of closeness to other members during this phase. Any missing members become a focus of discussion. Members will want to know, "Why isn't Mary here tonight?"

In some ways, when the group reaches this healing and growth phase, when it's doing its *work*, the group is (or seems like it is) on autopilot. However, this is not a reason for the leader to withdraw from their role. The group needs direction and guidance to achieve the working stage, just like an orchestra needs a conductor to make beautiful music.

And also remember that not every group meeting will go smoothly. Depending on the mix of group members you have, their mood, even the temperature of the room and the phase of the moon, the storm can return and you can have what you feel is a bad meeting. If this is the case, do not be discouraged! At this point in the group's progress, you can honestly and openly talk about challenges and turn breakdowns into breakthroughs. Don't forget to use a bit of humor too!

In sum, the working stage has allowed the group's members to be able to step outside of themselves and evaluate, accept, and even appreciate who they are and what they've done on the hard journey of caring for a loved one with dementia—thanks in large part to the interdependence of the group experience.

The primary leadership roles during this phase of growth and healing are similar to those of the prior phase and include:

- Continuing to model listening, openness, and caring.

- Being supportive of continued participation of group members.

- Being responsive to conflicts, resistance, or other problems that might arise (some storming can still occur during the working stage).

- Encouraging communication between group members by using the skills of facilitating, linking, and initiating (refer back to the basic skills section).

- Allowing and encouraging the group to be more self-responsible.

- Making appropriate adjustments to content and format based on the direction the group wants to go or is taking itself.

- When appropriate, letting the group know their last meeting together is coming next week (preparing them for closure)

- PHASE FIVE (closing):
Preparation for and leaving the group
When a support group has progressed through the prior four phases, when they've done their forming, storming, norming, and working, having achieved a certain level of intimacy, there will naturally be feelings of separation anxiety as they anticipate the group's end and the feelings of loss they may experience as they disperse and go

their own ways. It's possible that the support group is so successful that members will resist the ending. However, "graduation" from the support group is an important step for members. They've learned what their eight central needs are as dementia care partners. They've learned about the brain, behavior challenges in their loved one and how to respond to them, grief and loss, self-care and wellness, getting more help, and legal, financial, and end-of-life issues. They've asked the difficult "why" and "how" questions. And now, better equipped for what's ahead, with new friends at their side and resources in their hip pocket, they must move ahead on the journey down a path not chosen. And who better to launch them than their group leader and their fellow group mates?

Expect a certain amount of ambiguity of feelings about the ending of the group. Ending may elicit withdrawal in some, sadness in others, and happiness in yet others. A theme of general optimism and feelings of growth and healing should override any natural feelings of loss. The group leader must be sensitive to any and all feelings connected to members leaving the group, but at the same time, they can be proud that they have effectively and compassionately led this group toward integration. The last lesson in *The Dementia Care-Partner's Workbook* is very intentional in facilitating a meaningful and healthy closing stage to the ten-week curriculum.

Primary leadership roles during this last phase include:

- Recognizing and understanding the dynamics that occur as the group comes to an end.
- Encouraging reflection on individual and group growth related to the dementia care-partnering journey.
- Creating safe opportunities for members to say goodbye to each other and to the group.
- Providing counseling referrals and/or additional resources to those in need.
- Conducting an evaluation of the group.

In closing, a reminder: This five-phase theoretical model will be influenced by the unique personalities of your group members as well as by the style of the leaders. Some groups will move more slowly or quickly through some phases rather than others. The most important thing you can do as group leader is to ask yourself how you can make it safe for these phases to evolve. If your group is not moving forward, seems to be stuck, or is even going backward, try to discern why the members don't feel a sense of trust or safety. We'll talk more about this in the next section.

Challenges in the group

Murphy's Law ensures that no dementia care-partner support group will run smoothly 100 percent of the time. Problems will arise. In the second phase (the storming stage), they are even to be expected.

Here are some of the more common reasons and challenges to consider when things don't seem to be going right in the group.

Lack of leader preparation and/or training. "Where are we supposed to meet?" "How long was this meeting supposed to last?" "I thought *you* were going to bring the name tags!" If administrative details aren't properly planned for and executed, group members will feel left in the lurch. On the other hand, problems can also arise related to the leader's personality, skills, or training. An over-controlling or weak leader can stifle a group's progress or leave a group floundering. A lack of effective leadership skills can also impact a group's progress. For example, leaders who do not understand the group's basic needs, or who are not well-versed in basic counseling skills, may not be able to usher the group through its five developmental phases. Proper support-group leader training will circumvent these problems.

Discrepancies between group members' expectations and leader's expectations. Each individual group member will have their own expectations for the group. When a member's expectations haven't been met, they will usually respond in one of two ways—either by withdrawing from the group (by communicating their disappointment and letting the leader know they won't be coming any longer, or just not showing up), or by being very vocal in group and airing their gripes about failed expectations. There are several ways to mitigate unmet expectations. The first is provide as much information as possible about the group during the advertising of the group, through flyers or brochures, for example. Second, prescreening potential group members provides an opportunity to let people know what to expect of the group and let them share their goals for being part of the group process. Third, during the first meeting (the forming stage), review the guidelines and allow group members to have input and react to them. For leaders, it's important to realize that some expression of disappointment about you, the curriculum, or the group is normal (especially during the storming stage) and that by the group's end, much of the angst has often resolved.

Challenging members. Each person brings a unique personality and history to the group. No matter how well you prescreen members, you are likely to encounter challenging members who will test the skills of even the most skilled and experienced group leader. The most effective way to manage challenging members and situations is to foster, as group leader, a caring, trusting relationship between yourself and each group member. Sometimes group members will themselves intervene by confronting each other about the problems that have arisen in the group.

The following are descriptions of some of the more common challenging folks you as group leader are likely to encounter when leading dementia care-partner support groups. Suggestions are provided with each example as ways you might deal with them, but keep in mind that confronting an individual member in front of the rest of the group is rarely a good idea. Instead, ask to meet with them individually after the meeting, or, if there is a great deal of emotion, have the co-leader step out with the person who is upset (this is one of the best and most important reasons to have a co-leader). And remember, even when you must confront, lead with your heart, use your supportive listening skills, and respond with compassion and understanding. Usually, challenging members are just teaching you about their personalities and their unique ways of interacting with others.

- **Amy the Absent**

  Amy is the group member who is there, but is not there. Sometimes this person is a relatively new care partner and is still in shock over their loved one's dementia diagnosis. She is simply unable to speak yet. Amy may have tried to attend the support group too soon, or she may just need the group to be patient and understanding. However, there are also Amys who consciously choose not to participate and interact with the group in passive-aggressive ways: "I'm here, but I don't plan to be a part of this group." In Lesson Ten of *The Dementia Care-Partner's Workbook*, I tell the story of Sue Ann, a reluctant support-group member who was an Amy the Absent in the first few group meetings.

  Appropriate ways to intervene: From the very first meeting on, make an effort to help everyone feel involved and a part of the group. Create safe ways to invite the Amys in, such as asking, "Amy, I'm wondering what your week has been like since we met last?" Making eye contact even when this person is quiet is also a way of engaging her and inviting her participation. If your Amy is an outright passive-aggressive, you may need to talk to her individually and explore whether the group can appropriately meet her needs at this time. You may discover that some people are just very shy, quiet, or overwhelmed—yet they perceive they are getting a lot out of the group experience. The group is usually aware of who the Amys are, and can often embrace and accept their quiet nature and usually gentle spirit.

- **Ann the Advice-Giver**

  Even though you have created a ground rule that says, "Do not give advice unless it is asked for," you will, no doubt, have an Ann in one of your groups at some point. Ann is quick to inform others what they should do to solve problems. She may try to "take over" under the guise of being helpful.

Appropriate ways to intervene: Gently remind Ann of the ground rule about advice-giving, or ask, "Did you feel that John needed you to tell him what to do about his concerns?" Obviously, the goal is to prevent advice-giving in your group unless it is asked for.

- **Albert the Academic**
  Albert is the intellectual in the group and often likes to show off his huge knowledge base. He might quote a recent article he read or expose a little-known theory to explain something about the biology or progression of dementia, for example. Analysis and interpretation are Albert's joys in life! There may be a condescending quality to his tone; generally he thinks he knows more than most anyone else in the group.

  Appropriate ways to intervene: Initially, Albert needs to feel part of the group like any others member. However, when his intellectualizing becomes a consistent pattern, especially if it is condescending, it can be destructive to the group. It can be helpful to say something like, "Albert, you have really helped us understand this topic more, but I do wonder how you *feel*." Of course, he may lack insight, but it is worth a try. If you as group leader have a strong relationship with Albert, you could say, "Albert, I know that I sometimes have a tendency to intellectualize things that are painful for me. I wonder if you see that same tendency in yourself?"

- **Bob the Blamer**
  Bob is the member who projects that other group members (or other people in general) are the ones who cause his problems. This self-defeating thought pattern has often been a part of his coping mechanisms for some time. Bobs often projects an accompanying sense that no one has ever understood him and no one ever will. This self-crippling stance wears thin very quickly with members who are trying to honestly look at themselves and sort out new directions in

their lives. Sometimes Bob will see himself as having the solution to everyone else's problems. Bobs tend to take on one of three stances — blamer or victim most commonly, or, on occasion, rescuer.

Appropriate ways to intervene: Compassionately attempt to help Bob become more self-responsible and eliminate the tendency to blame. Well-timed, tentative comments like, "Bob, sometimes I'm struck by how often you find fault with others. I'm wondering what would happen for you if you looked inside yourself at times instead of outside?" A supportive confrontation like this has the potential of getting Bob more connected to himself and starts to help him make positive changes.

- **Charlene the Challenging**
Charlene is the member who likes to challenge the leader. She might accuse the leader of not knowing what they are saying or doing, which in turn may cause the leader, especially an inexperienced or untrained one, to question themselves. Charlene likes to put leaders on the spot and tries to make them look incompetent in the eyes of the group. Her challenges are more often made in front of the group than privately.

Appropriate ways to intervene: As a leader, be certain you don't get defensive when Charlene's challenges are forthcoming. This may be just what she wants (consciously or unconsciously) and would probably lead to more conflict and confrontation. It is often appropriate to acknowledge her comment but then offer to meet her after the group to better understand each other. While you may be tempted to initiate a dialogue that will prove your competence, resist the urge. The group will most often respect your decision to deflect the criticism and discuss the situation individually with Charlene rather than bear witness to an argument or battle of wits.

- **Fred the Forced**
Fred is the group member who is there because someone else wants him there. He has no intention of participating and feels he has been

forced into coming by a family member or friend. He hopes everyone will forget he is present and will leave him alone. Fred rarely makes eye contact with anyone, particularly the group leader. If questioned or invited to participate, he often passes and looks put upon.

Appropriate ways to intervene: Fred is the kind of person you as leader would want to prevent from joining the group through the prescreening process because he will be counterproductive if not outright damaging to the group. Once Fred is in the group, though, you can attempt to make him feel welcome and warmly invite his participation. However, if that doesn't work, the group will be well-served if you meet with Fred individually and explore the possibility of him leaving the group. You may also consider referring Fred for individual counseling, but he will usually resist this suggestion.

- **Holly the Holy Roller**
Holly spends so much time talking about heaven that people wonder if her feet are on the ground! While spirituality is a very important part of group and should be explored (in fact, Lesson Nine focuses on existential and spiritual issues), the Hollys of the group often alienate other members by imposing their beliefs on everyone else in the group to the exclusion or unacceptance of other belief systems. Hollys usually projects a lack of any personal problems and may perceive other members' caregiving challenges as a "lack of faith."

Appropriate ways to intervene: As leader, you can accept how important Holly's faith is to her, help others in the group acknowledge that faith and spirituality are of comfort to many, but also support the notion that what works for one person may not work for another. If Holly is advice-giving about the need for everyone to have faith like hers, you must gently remind her of the ground rules and redirect the group in ways supportive to everyone present.

- **Ivan the Interrupter**
Ivan is the group member who, whether he's aware of it or not, is always interrupting other people. He can't seem to keep his mouth

shut. Other members will begin to see it coming and will start hesitating to share for fear they will be interrupted. Ivan must be helped to control his interrupting tendencies or he will damage the very heart of the group.

Appropriate ways to intervene: Gently remind Ivan of the "equal time" ground rule. When this fails, go to the next step: "Ivan, I notice that sometimes you have a tendency to interrupt the person who is talking. Are you aware of this?" Or, "Ivan, what you have to say is important, but let's hear from some others who haven't had a chance to share today." Sometimes I will sit by an Ivan when in group. A gentle hand on his arm when he is getting ready to interrupt, even with a whisper of something true but humorous ("Here you go again"), can be helpful.

- **Paul the Preacher/Teacher**
Paul has a lot in common with Holly, but he often preaches and teaches about anything and everything. The group experience provides Paul with an audience. He may attempt to dominate the group as he tells them what they should and should not do, what they need or must know. He is usually very well-intentioned but tends to wear thin with the group. He may seem overly rehearsed, as if he has preached his message many times.

Appropriate ways to intervene: Gently remind Paul of the "equal time" ground rule, as well as the "advice-giving" ground rule. As leader, you may want to talk with Paul before or after the meeting, expressing how his constant tendency to preach and teach impacts *you*. Say, for example, "Sometimes when I listen to you, Paul, I wonder if you really want to hear what others think and feel." Again, this confrontation must be well-timed and intended to help him reflect on how he is impacting the group.

- **Ralph the Rambler**
Ralph is a close cousin of Paul the Preacher/Teacher—he just changes subjects more often. Ralph tends to bore the group as he rambles on,

yet seems to say little of substance related to the needs of the group. He rarely completes his sentences in ways that allow others to talk; he just keeps running on and on and on. The group kind of lets out a silent groan as soon as Ralph utters his first words. Without a doubt, one rambling Ralph can short-circuit a group if there is not an effective intervention.

Appropriate ways to intervene: Once again, return to the ground rules related to "equal time." If this fails, step up your efforts to help Ralph by being supportively direct about his tendency to talk a lot. The group will often be able to help if you ask them if anyone was able to follow what Ralph just said. There is some risk in this approach in that a fellow group member may attack Ralph for rambling on all the time and saying little. Again, if all else fails, ask to speak with Ralph after the meeting and attempt to compassionately help him look at his rambling and become a more controlled contributor to the group.

- **Sarah the Socializer**
  Sarah's goal is to keep the group from getting too serious about anything. The problem here, of course, is that a dementia diagnosis in a loved one and being an isolated and stressed care partner will naturally bring about serious, thoughtful, and often painful discussions. Sarah may see the group as an opportunity to be with other people and socialize in a fun way. Obviously, her expectations are different than the group's. Sarah may laugh when everyone else is sad or make inappropriate comments to distract the group from the work at hand.

  Appropriate ways to intervene: First, understand that many people protect themselves from getting hurt by trying to stay in a social mode or be humorous. Freud recognized humor as one of our ego defense mechanisms over a century ago. Try well-timed, sensitive comments like, "I notice that sometimes you laugh when others are sad. What do you think about that?" Or, "When I see you laugh like that, I wonder what you are really feeling?" Some Sarahs will lack insight into their use of socializing, while others will allow you to penetrate the veneer of humor and access deeper feelings of anxiety, worry, or fear, and appreciate your efforts to try to help them.

- **Wally the We-Sayer**
Wally attempts to talk for everyone in the group or to be the group spokesperson. "We think we should . . ." is a common lead for this person. Wally assumes (and this is what creates problems) that everyone thinks and feels the same as he does. Allowing the "we" messages to continue often causes quieter members to give in to the "we talk" Wally espouses. Resentment can arise, disrupting the group's growth and even causing members to question whether they want to continue participating.

Appropriate ways to intervene: Gently confronting Wally by asking if he is speaking for every person in the group or asking the group if there is anyone who doesn't agree with his statement may be an effective way to manage Wally's we-saying. If you have a healthy, well-functioning group, members will feel free to express themselves, agreeing or disagreeing with Wally. If done in a supportive manner, Wally's we-saying can be integrated into the group and recognized as one of many unique personalities present. If necessary, meeting with Wally separately can also be helpful.

Determining when a group member needs individual counseling and asking a group member to leave the group.
Even when prescreening group members has occurred, once in a while it will turn out that a member isn't suited to participating in the group and will need to be asked to leave. If this has happened to you as a group leader, no worries! Even the most prepared, well-trained, and experienced leaders can misjudge a person who seems to be a perfect fit for group but turns out not to be.

When you discover there is a mismatch between a member's needs and the group's ability to help, as group leader you have an ethical responsibility to ask the person to leave the group and refer them to other sources of support and care. It doesn't mean the person cannot return to the group at a later time, it just means now is not the best time for them to be a member. This usually happens when a member is in crisis, has serious mental-health challenges, feels overwhelmed and over their head, or their personality challenges are so great that despite remediation, they just don't fit in. Despite your best intentions, the group cannot meet this person's needs, and the group will suffer if they are forced to spend the bulk of their time on this one member to the exclusion of everyone else.

The bottom line is that it's inappropriate to try to care for someone in a support *group* who really needs professional *individual* counseling. In a case like this, an appropriate referral should be made, and typically, the person on the receiving end of the referral recognizes they need more help and is grateful. You should be knowledgeable about your community's therapists and their areas of specialty so that you can make the best possible referral.

Here are some "red flags" that a member of the support group needs an individual counselor (or in cases of extreme distress, hospitalization) and that dismissal from the group and a referral are necessary. They are:

- Persistent thoughts of suicide, expressions of serious suicide intent, or the development of a specific suicide plan
- Arriving to group under the influence of alcohol or drugs
- Previous diagnosis of a serious mental-health disorder
- Profound symptoms of anxiety or depression that interfere with the ability to do basic self-care
- Uncontrollable anger and rage directed at the leader or other members
- Uncontrollable anxiety, worry, fear, or guilt that prevents active participation in the group
- Physical harm to self or others
- Uncontrollable phobias

Please note, this list is not all-inclusive. Judgment should be used as to whether or not a group member would benefit more from individual counseling than from a support group. It is also important for leaders to realize that, even when you make a referral for individual counseling, the person may choose not to take your advice.

When the group just doesn't seem to be going well and you're not sure why.

Over the last 12 years, I've led many support groups of varying types, including pregnancy and infant-loss, loss of parent, spouse, or child, and of course dementia care-partner support groups. The vast majority of these groups went really well, but some were just OK, and a few didn't go well at all.

For the groups that were "duds," it can be hard to pinpoint exactly what went wrong. But if you're stuck in a foundering group, here are a couple of possible reasons why:

- **The leaders aren't doing their job well or don't work well together.** As you've read so many times thus far in *A Leader's Manual*, the choice of who leads (and co-leads) the support group is the most important step in the planning process. If the leader(s) aren't passionate about the topic, or are ambivalent about leading, unprepared, and/or lack training and skills, even the best curriculum won't help.

- **The members don't mix well together.** Even with great planning, including prescreening potential members, and even in the absence of overtly challenging members like the ones described, sometimes the individuals who make up the group don't mix well together. Perhaps it's related to a lack of trust (in the leaders, or that confidentiality won't be maintained, or for some other reason). Maybe members are unwilling to self-disclose and/or be vulnerable. I had one group with mostly Alzheimer's care partners but several whose loved ones had behavioral variant frontotemporal dementia. Early on, one of them said, "There is no way you (meaning the

Alzheimer's care partners) can understand what I'm going through." She and the other FTD care partners decided they weren't going to benefit, yet they stayed till the end and the group as a whole just never "clicked."

When a group doesn't make progress for whatever reason(s), they don't cycle through the five phases of support groups naturally. They get stuck, usually in the forming and especially the storming stage, without norming and working, so that as leader, you find yourself having to close the group in week ten not feeling a sense of accomplishment. Though feeling discouraged about this would be a normal reaction, wait to see how members assess their group experience in the end-of-group evaluation forms. Members often rate their experience better than you'd expect.

No matter how you perceive the group is going, or went, whatever the case may be, keep in mind the following: You did work through the ten lessons of *The Dementia Care-Partner's Workbook*, members were exposed to the eight central needs of dementia care partners (even if they haven't addressed them all), you as leader valued, respected, and heard each and every individual in the group, and most likely, members developed better coping mechanisms, learned new skills, and developed some resilience.

Perhaps you as leader have to "trust the process," just as you ask your members to do!

When a group member or their loved one with dementia dies

It is likely, if you lead enough dementia care-partner support groups, that at some point a care partner in the group or more likely the loved one with dementia of a participating care partner will die. Caregiving is, after all, stressful, and dementia is an incurable disease. This can be challenging for the group leader and members of the group to deal with. If a group member dies, the leader should share this information with the others in a sensitive and compassionate manner, taking as much time as needed to understand and process what happened and letting group members grieve for their comrade and fellow journeyer. Organizing a group card or flowers for the family may be a helpful way for the group to mourn the loss. If the loved one of a group member dies from their dementia, I typically invite the care partner to come back for one meeting, to allow that person to share the final chapter of their loved one's story and to let others express their condolences.

Meeting Plans For
Lessons One Through Ten
OF THE DEMENTIA CARE-PARTNER'S WORKBOOK

A few introductory words for leaders before jumping into meeting plans

We have all probably heard the cliché "location, location, location" when it comes to success in real estate. You've heard many times what I am now going to repeat when it comes to leading a successful dementia care-partner support group: "planning, planning, planning." In other words, don't try to "wing it"!

I know that some of you using *A Leader's Manual* will be tempted to go straight to this section, skim the meeting plan, and "jump in." I would strongly discourage you from taking this approach. Each of the ten lessons in *The Dementia Care-Partner's Workbook* is chockfull of information and questions. You will need to be thoroughly familiar with each lesson's content, as well as the meeting plan, to lead effectively. There is enough information in each lesson, particularly lessons two through eight, to expand the number of meetings to more than ten if desired. In addition, the meeting plans, while unique to each of the ten lessons, can be modified as you see fit; what I've outlined is intended as a suggestion. Be creative and consider adding some of your own activities if that would best meet the needs of your unique group. I have created an overview of the ten weekly meetings to provide a snapshot of the corresponding lesson in the *Workbook*, educational topics, and discussion questions (Appendix 4) to assist with the planning process.

Please note that during the first meeting, you should be prepared to pass out copies of *The Dementia Care-Partner's Workbook* to each member. You can order the books through Companion Press (www. centerforloss.com). If you are ordering in bulk, you may be eligible for a discounted price. Contact the publisher at (970) 226-6050 or www. centerforloss.com for more information.

A few words about members doing homework

As I said in the prior section, each of the ten lessons in *The Dementia Care-Partner's Workbook* is loaded with lots of information. The content of each lesson has been carefully chosen to inform dementia care partners about everything they need to know from diagnosis and the beginning of the journey all the way to the late stage and the end of the journey. Depending on where a care partner's loved one is, some of the information may or may not be applicable to them. Ideally, care partners would read ahead and complete the journaling in the *Workbook* prior to coming to the meeting covering that lesson. In my experience, some group members will faithfully do their homework, and some will not. Whether they are too busy, too stressed, or just too tired, some will participate in meetings without having prepared. They will still benefit from the group experience and what's covered in each meeting, and will refer back to the *Workbook* as needed in the future.

Anatomy of a meeting plan

If you plan to do baseline and end-of-group assessments

On pages 16 to 17 of *A Leader's Manual*, I described a number of assessments you can use with your group members at baseline (prior to Meeting One) and at the end (during or after Meeting Ten). The most common of these are the Zarit Caregiver Burden Scale, the Geriatric Depression Scale, and the Geriatric Anxiety Scale, among others.

If you wish to do baseline assessments, I would suggest sending the assessment forms to members ahead of time with a cover letter explaining what they're for and asking them to bring the completed forms to the first meeting. This will save precious group time. Bring some extra printouts to the first meeting in case some members didn't get them or forgot. You can send them home and ask them to bring them to the second meeting. As I'll explain in the Meeting Ten plan, you can take a few minutes to have members complete the end-of-group assessments during group time. That way you'll have them in hand.

Before the group begins
Plan to meet your co-leader at the meeting room an hour before group starts. You'll want to go ahead and set up chairs in the room first. Depending on the size and shape of the room, you'll arrange the chairs in a circle or oval. It's important that all members are sitting together, so that each member can easily see and make eye contact with all other members, you, and your co-leader. I like to sit on opposite sides of the circle/oval from my co-leader, with the co-leader closest to the door, in case a member needs to be escorted out of the room during the meeting.

Place a small table by the door and put name tags, markers, a small waste receptacle, a sign-in sheet, and any other flyers or brochures related to your organization or community services. Another table or area should be designated for drinks and snacks. You and your co-leader can decide what to serve. At a minimum, coffee, water, cookies, and cheese and/or peanut butter crackers are appreciated by all. You can even ask group members to take turns bringing snacks.

Once the room, chairs, and tables are set up, you and your co-leader should divide and conquer responsibilities for who will do what during the meeting. You can keep the same roles and responsibilities throughout all group meetings, or change it up. The latter is optimal if the co-leader will eventually go on to lead their own group.

Before group ("warm-up")
Members will start arriving to the group as much as 30 minutes before the starting time. You can decide when to open the doors to the actual

meeting room. If there is an area to wait outside the meeting room, I generally don't open the doors until 15 minutes before the group starts. I have found that certain members always come early to socialize with other members, or to have some one-on-one time with the co-leader or me. More quiet, introverted members may particularly like what I refer to as their before-group warm-up time. Sometimes the best counseling happens before the group even gets started!

Opening the group

It is important to have an official start to each weekly meeting. Try to start (and end) each meeting on time. Recognize that usually one or two members will be chronically late, but for the rest of the group, starting on time demonstrates your respect for their time. Some dementia care partners have very little flexibility with their time. Their loved one may be home alone, or with a family member or friend who is watching them as a favor. Begin with a warm welcome (I'll go into the welcome for the first meeting in more detail in the next section). Let everyone know you're glad to see them. I usually remind the group what meeting and lesson we're on, what the topic of today's/tonight's meeting is, and how many meetings we have remaining before the group comes to an end. I'll then ask if anyone has a question or thought before we begin, then move on to the Mindfulness Moment. This part of group should take about five minutes.

Mindfulness Moment

Mindfulness is a component of each and every lesson in *The Dementia Care-Partner's Workbook*. A detailed explanation of what mindfulness is, and how we practice mindfulness, is provided in Lesson One of the *Workbook*. In the first few meetings, most members will find mindfulness to be an awkward experience. Older care partners, especially, may not be familiar with mindfulness and may equate it with an Eastern practice that they are concerned might be in conflict with their own spiritual or religious practices. Once they learn what it is, these apprehensions disappear, and by the third meeting, it often becomes the part members look forward to most. Of course, if you are working through *The Dementia Care-Partner's Workbook* in a faith-based setting, you may want to substitute or supplement the Mindfulness Moment with prayer, for example. The Mindfulness Moment is meant to be exactly that, just a moment. This part of the group should take about five minutes.

Check-in

Other than the first meeting, what occurs next is a vital activity for dementia care partners: check-in. It is my belief that every member in the group needs some talk time, even if they are apprehensive about being in a group, shy, or introverted. As I've mentioned, Central Need 1 of dementia care partners is to tell and retell their story. In essence, check-in is a brief telling of the part of their story that happened during the prior week.

I usually begin check-in with a brief, open-ended statement such as, "Let's take some time to see how your week has been since the last time we met." If you want to be a bit more directive, you could say, "Perhaps you'd be willing to share a success or challenge you've had this past week." Another approach is this: "Last week we talked about the lobes of the brain and what each of them does. Did you find this information was helpful to you during the last week?" You will likely find the question that best suits you and your leadership style when leading check-in.

Check-in should last no more than one-third the length of your group, so for a 90-minute meeting, check-in would be up to 30 minutes, typically 15 to 20. If it is any longer than that, you may run out of time to do the other components of each meeting. However, use your judgment. Sometimes check-in needs to last longer, especially during the norming and working stages of the group. In order to keep check-in at the desired length, you'll have to do some quick math just before it begins. If you have ten members, they'd each have about three minutes to check in. Let everyone know how long they have to check in, and don't be afraid to politely cut someone off when their time is up. They will get used to you doing this.

Education

Each of the ten lessons in *The Dementia Care-Partner's Workbook* has an educational component that covers several related topics as well as Central Needs. There is a lot of content in each lesson, more than you could possibly cover in one meeting. You'll need to decide what you want to emphasize in this part of each meeting, and assume or hope members will learn the rest on their own. Plan to spend about 15 to 20 minutes on the educational content, either all at once or broken into two or three segments associated with the related discussion question(s). You won't necessarily be covering it verbatim from the *Workbook*, of course, but you may choose to hit the highlights, or prepare a synopsis of the topic(s) you want to review. In some cases, depending on your experience, interest, or area of expertise, you may want to cover a topic in more detail and share that with the group. The educational content you review should revolve around the discussion question(s) you want the group to talk about in the next part of the meeting.

Note that you don't have to be an expert in all the areas of content you present or review. If you've read the entire lesson from beginning to end, and looked up concepts that you don't understand or want more information on (see Resources section at the back of the *Workbook*), you'll know more than most members, and if you don't know the answer to a question, you can always look it up for the next meeting or suggest the care partner ask their loved one's healthcare provider.

Discussion

The Dementia Care-Partner's Workbook is full of stories and questions with space for the reader to do some journaling related to the educational content. The discussion should take at or just over a third of the total time for the group, about 30 to 40 minutes for a 90-minute meeting. Select two or three questions that you wish to discuss, starting with the one you most want to have the group discuss first.

Or, you may want to discuss the group's reaction to one of the stories. Spend ten to 15 minutes on each question/story, and do your best, over the 30 to 40 minutes, to encourage each member to share something at least once, by calling on members if necessary. If you have a large group of 12 or more members, and you have the space to do it, you can break the group in half for the discussion, so that you take half and your co-leader takes the other half. Or, if half your members are spouses/partners, the other half adult children, you could divide the group by care-partner type. It's OK to try breakout groups one week to see how it goes. The advantage is more opportunity for members to share; the downside is that it can disrupt group unity and cohesion.

Preview of next meeting and homework

If everything up until this point goes as planned, there should be about ten minutes left in the meeting following the discussion. Tell the group you're beginning the wrap-up. Remind them which lesson in the *Workbook* is up next, and encourage them to read ahead and journal their responses if they wish. Though some dementia care partners will be too busy to do homework, others will read every lesson in advance and complete written responses to all the questions. The group becomes a lifeline for them.

Mindfulness Moment

If there is time, you may want to close the group with another Mindfulness Moment. For many care partners, their only downtime in the week may be the Mindfulness Moments at the beginning and end of group. However, if you've run out of time, you can skip the closing Mindfulness Moment and encourage members to engage mindfully before they go to bed tonight and again in the morning when they wake up.

Closing

As the group members are preparing to leave, thank them for coming and participating. Remind them that the next meeting will be in one week, same time, same place. Just as you intentionally welcomed everyone at the beginning, officially dismiss them for the evening. Try to be on time with dismissal. If you do run over, don't be bothered if some care partners go ahead and leave. They probably have special arrangements for the care of their loved one during group.

After group ("afterburn")

I am always amazed by the number of people who linger after the end of group, mostly to talk to one another (many great conversations have occurred in the parking lot), but sometimes, to meet with my co-leader or me for an "afterburn" discussion. I try to make myself available for 15 minutes after group ends for those who remain behind for some one-on-one time. After the 15 minutes is up, I will usually tell them I need to work with the co-leader to return the room to its original condition, and dismiss them for the night with a fond farewell. I feel this is another important boundary to set.

Leader and co-leader decompression time

After everyone has left, as you and your co-leader are breaking the room down and putting things away, it is important to have a time when the two of you decompress and discuss how you felt the meeting went. This may only take 10 or 15 minutes, but it's very important, especially if you are an experienced leader and have a lay leader or student as co-leader, in which case it becomes a time of teaching and learning. It's also important for your own self-care. Talk about how you feel the meeting went by doing a shortened SWOT analysis (strengths-weaknesses-opportunities-threats). You will likely want to talk about specific group members, especially challenging ones and how you might approach them next week in the group. You might want to do some preplanning for the next week, especially if you like to divide and conquer the education and discussion times.

MEETING ONE

TELLING YOUR STORY FROM THE BEGINNING

Note: Review the Appendix 4 overview and the previous section "Anatomy of a meeting plan" for information relevant to all meetings.

Meeting overview and key topics

In this first meeting of the ten-week support group, your overarching goal will be to make members feel welcome and safe. You can station yourself near the door to direct people, ask them to sign in (for this first sign-in, provide space for them to write their email address, phone number, and whether they give permission to share their contact information with other group members), make a name tag (make sure you and your co-leader have one too), grab a drink and snack, then sit down. Your co-leader can be stationed in the middle of the circle, directing people where to sit. Each of you can introduce yourselves as you greet and assist people. The first meeting always feels a bit chaotic.

Opening

Begin by welcoming everyone to the group. Acknowledge that they may be feeling anxious and uncertain, and normalize these feelings. Introduce yourself by telling them a bit about you and your family, what you do professionally, perhaps your hobbies or things you like to do outside work, and why you've chosen to lead the group. Then have your co-leader do the same.

Next you can pass out everyone's copy of *The Dementia Care-Partner's Workbook*. I would also suggest you provide a printed schedule with the dates the ten weekly meetings will be held and the *Workbook* lesson number and chapter title that will be covered each week. Include the time the group will start and end, as well as the location name and address. You can also provide your contact information on the schedule if you wish (in case members are ill or can't come, and want to let you know).

Next you will talk about the structure of the group meetings. Go over the schedule. Remind them tonight is different because it's the initial meeting, but in general, you will start on time and end on time, open the room 15 minutes before group starts, and stay a few minutes after to answer questions. If you're meeting during the winter months and anticipate bad weather on a day you're meeting, either provide a number they can call to see if group is canceled, or use the email/phone list on the sign-in sheet to alert them the group won't be meeting. Describe the flow of each 90-minute meeting: beginning with a Mindfulness Moment (which they'll experience shortly), then check-in, an educational lesson, discussion questions, and a reminder of what's ahead for the following week.

Next you can share a bit about the organization of *The Dementia Care-Partner's Workbook*. Have them turn to page 10 of the Introduction and skim over the names of each of the ten lessons. You can tell them that each lesson contains a lot of information, more than you'll be able to cover in 90 minutes, but it's there for them to read and digest as homework or at their own pace. Then have them turn to page 7 of the Introduction to tell them about the eight central needs of dementia care partners. You can have them take turns reading each of the needs aloud. Then share that each weekly lesson will cover several topics and one or several of the central needs.

This would also be a good time to talk about journaling. Mention that each lesson has a number of questions that follow individual sections of the educational content. Space is provided for journaling. On page 11 of the Introduction, there is a text box describing the benefits of journaling, which you can briefly summarize if you wish. This is a good time to acknowledge that some people are more inclined to journal than others, but for the reasons you just mentioned, journaling is generally a helpful thing to do, and you encourage them to give it a try.

Whether or not members journal in advance of each meeting, ask them to bring the *Workbook* to every meeting.

Next you will go over the ground rules (see Appendix 1; feel free to modify the sample ground rules included with *A Leader's Manual* to meet your needs). You may want to pass out one or two copies of the ground rules per person and ask them to sign one copy and return it to you and keep a copy for themselves. Give a few sentences of background as to why ground rules are important, and that you may refer back to them from time to time in the weeks ahead. Then you can read the ground rules aloud or have members take turns reading them. Afterward, emphasize the ground rule on confidentiality and any others you see fit. From welcoming everyone to going over the ground rules, this part of the meeting should take about 30 minutes.

Mindfulness Moment

Now comes the time for the very first Mindfulness Moment. Have members open their books to Lesson One, page 20. Read the description of mindfulness from the text on pages 20 to 21, then lead the group through the breathing exercise. If mindfulness is new to you, practice with your co-leader before the group begins so you're familiar with the routine. This first Mindfulness Moment will take ten minutes or so, but in future meetings, it will usually be just five.

Check-in

Instead of a typical weekly check-in, you will use the time in this first meeting for group members to introduce themselves. Begin with these instructions: "We will now take time for each of you to briefly introduce yourselves to the other members of the group. Take a couple of minutes each and tell us your name, something about your family, who your loved one is who has dementia and what type of dementia they have, and how long you have been their care partner." You'll want to limit this time to 30 minutes, so each member will have just two to three minutes each. As members introduce themselves, I always write down each member's name, their spouse/partner's name, diagnosis, and how long ago they were diagnosed (keep this list handy for future reference—group members like and appreciate when you call them and their loved one with dementia by name). If they go beyond this time, interrupt them, thank them for sharing, and say something like, "We'll look forward to getting to know you even better in future weeks."

Education and discussion

Normally, the education and discussion components of group are done separately, and take up the most time. The first week is unique in this regard. At this point you will only have about 20 minutes left.

Go back to page 7 of the Introduction and read the paragraph on Central Need 1—Tell and retell your story. Then ask the question that's on page 25 of Lesson One: "How and when did your loved one begin to experience symptoms of dementia?" If you want, you or someone in the group can read out loud about the early symptoms of my late wife Rebecca's early-onset Alzheimer's disease to give them an idea of what to share, but this isn't necessary. You will have time for several group members to share about their loved one's initial symptoms. Or if you'd like, ask the question: "Tell the group what your loved one's first symptom of dementia was," which will allow everyone to briefly share.

If for some reason not everyone was able to introduce themselves during the check-in time, you could ask those who didn't to do so now, and have them share their loved one's diagnosis and first symptom of dementia. When you see there are just five minutes left, transition to the preview and closing.

Preview and closing

For the end of the first meeting, you'll do a quick review then preview before closing. Invite members to read the Introduction and Lesson One on their own before next week. Encourage them to journal. Most of the journaling questions in Lesson One are prompts for them to share different aspects of their loved one's diagnosis with dementia. Then read about next week's lesson on the bottom of page 32 and top of page 33. Encourage them to read the text box entitled "If You're Feeling Overwhelmed" on page 33. Also encourage them to read Lesson Two and answer those journaling questions as well. If you have time, you can repeat the Mindfulness Moment.

Before dismissing the class, tell them these three things: 1) Thank them for coming, 2) Tell them they may feel really tired physically and mentally after today's/tonight's meeting, and that this is normal, and 3) Gently warn them they may not want to come back next week, but please do, they'll be glad they did, because it's important to "trust the process."

Congratulations, you made it through the first meeting!

MEETING TWO

BASICS OF ALZHEIMER'S DISEASE AND OTHER DEMENTIAS

Note: Review the Appendix 4 overview and the previous section "Anatomy of a meeting plan" for information relevant to all meetings.

Meeting overview and key topics

In the *Workbook*, Lesson Two is the first of two content-rich lessons on the brain. In this chapter on the "basics," topics include what dementia is, how it is diagnosed, risk factors for developing dementia, and a description of the pre-dementia diagnosis mild cognitive impairment as well as the common forms of dementia (Alzheimer's, vascular, frontotemporal, and Lewy body).

Meeting Two has two critical components, the check-in and a group activity that I will call the "emotions exercise," both of which are described below. There is a lot if information provided in Lesson Two of *The Dementia Care-Partner's Workbook*, some of which you won't have time to cover. What's most important in this second meeting is that members again feel welcome and safe, begin feeling a sense of belonging to the group and that they will benefit from coming each week, and begin to process some of the emotions associated with being a dementia care partner. Educationally, they should come away with an understanding of several important things: what dementia is (and isn't—it's a neurodegenerative disease, not part of the normal aging process), that there are different forms of dementia (Alzheimer's disease being the most common), and that it's incorrect to say "Alzheimer's and dementia." If you can accomplish these things, Meeting Two will be a success!

Opening

Welcome everyone back to this week's meeting. Acknowledge that it may have been difficult for some to return. Many if not most people do not want to be in a dementia care-partner support group! If any members missed the first week, have them introduce themselves.

Mindfulness Moment

Ask members to turn to page 39 of *The Dementia-Care Partner's Workbook*. Read the description of the Mindfulness Moment out loud again, then lead the group through the breathing exercise. After this week, you'll just guide members through the breathing exercise without referring to the *Workbook* because it's the same each time.

Check-in

Although check-in is an important part of every weekly meeting, I think it is most important in the second week because of the processing that's done during this time. Ask members the following: "Let's begin our check-in time today with (name the person to your right). (Their name), tell us how your week has been? Did the last week bring any particular successes or challenges with (their loved one with dementia's name)? What was it like for you to be in the group last week?"

The member will key in on the question they most want to answer. Give each person a few minutes to respond, then continue around the oval/circle until you're done. Keep your basic counseling skills in mind as people are responding. You'll use all of them today/tonight and in the weeks ahead during check-in (and discussion). You may have your first encounter with a challenging personality in the group during this check-in time. The group is in the forming stage still, but if you see some conflict arising between you and a member, or among members, be aware that the storming has begun!

Education

As mentioned, there is a lot of educational content in the *Workbook*'s Lesson Two. For your educational discussion today, focus on two things: the definition of dementia (pages 43 to 44) and the symptoms of whatever dementia diagnoses the loved ones in your group have (pages 51 to 59). From last week's introductions and the list you made, you should know which diagnoses are represented in the group. Statistically speaking, Alzheimer's and vascular dementia will be the most common.

Read aloud the symptoms for the diagnoses you'll be covering (Appendix 6 is a summary of the symptoms of the four most common forms of dementia in a checklist form, which you can hand out to your group members for this part of the meeting). It is likely that at least some members will have an "aha" moment as they hear a symptom that their loved one is experiencing that they hadn't previously attributed to the disease (this will be the first of many "aha" moments members will experience in group). If your group is comprised solely of members whose loved ones have Alzheimer's disease, don't feel compelled to review the symptoms of the other forms of dementia.

If the educational component only lasts ten to 15 minutes today, that's OK. Check-in and discussion are longer than normal in Meeting Two.

Discussion

For the discussion, you will begin with one of my favorite activities in *The Dementia Care-Partner's Workbook*, the emotions exercise.

Have members turn to page 37 in Lesson Two. Read through the introductory section in the text box entitled "Understanding Our Emotions." More than 70 emotions are listed on pages 37 and 38. They are also listed on a handout (Appendix 7). Each person will circle all the emotions they're feeling at present, but then select the *one* emotion they are feeling the most in response to their loved one's dementia. Have them write down why they chose this particular emotion (they may have already done this in their *Workbook* if they did homework), which they will then share with the group. Gauge the remaining time and allow each member their allotted time to share about the emotion they chose. In my experience, the most commonly chosen emotion is guilt, but responses can and do vary. When time is up, you may sense a difference in the closeness of group members to one another. This exercise usually gives the group a sense of unity and bonds them together.

If you have time remaining after the emotions exercise, you can have members share their loved one's symptoms from the Appendix 6 checklist, or ask if any members have questions from reading through either Lesson One or Lesson Two.

Preview and closing

If you have time and want to have an end-of-meeting Mindfulness Moment, please do so. Otherwise, tell the group members you will be covering the *Workbook*'s Lesson Three next week, a continuation of their study of the brain. A brief description of that lesson is provided in Lesson Two on the bottom of page 60 and the top of page 61, which you can read out loud if you wish. They'll learn about the brain lobes and what they do, the cognitive (memory and thinking) functions, activities of daily living, and the stages of dementia. Wish everyone well, then dismiss the group. Two meetings down, eight to go!

MEETING THREE

**BRAIN STRUCTURE AND FUNCTION,
ACTIVITIES OF DAILY LIVING, AND DEMENTIA STAGES**

*Note: Review the Appendix 4 overview and the previous section "Anatomy
of a meeting plan" for information relevant to all meetings.*

Meeting overview and key topics

In the *Workbook*, Lesson Three is jam-packed with information
about the brain, including a description of the four major brain lobes
and what their functions are, a description of the five cognitive
functions, cognitive-function testing, the definition of instrumental
and basic activities of daily living, the stages of dementia, from mild
cognitive impairment to early-, middle-, and late-stage dementia, and
medications used to treat dementia. This information, along with
Lesson Two on what dementia is and the different types of dementia,
address Central Need 2—Educate yourself (about the brain). There is
enough material in Lesson Three that it could easily be covered over
two or even three weeks. So much to learn, so little time!

Having led groups through this lesson content many times, the most
important thing many care partners learn from all the "brain stuff"
is that their loved one is further along in their dementia journey
than they thought. By learning about the stages, they also are struck
by what lies ahead for their loved one, no matter what stage they
are in now. The late stage of dementia is by far the most physically,
emotionally, and spiritually challenging for care partners, and they
realize this when they see the list of symptoms associated with it.
Because it would be nice to be able to work through two questions in

the discussion section, the opening, Mindfulness Moment, and check-in are intentionally brief for this week.

Opening and Mindfulness Moment

By now group members are used to you opening with a brief "welcome" and moving into the Mindfulness Moment. Today you can go straight to the breathing exercise without reading the description of what mindfulness is. Both these things should take about five minutes.

Check-in

Though check-in should be kept brief for this meeting, don't skip it. You never know when someone has had a particular high- or low-point in their week that they want and need to share with the group.

You can structure the check-in a couple of different ways in order to keep it short. For example, you might say: "Let's take time for a quick check-in. Who from the group would like to share a particular success or challenge from the past week?" Or, you could say: "Let's go around the circle and have everyone share one word that represents how their last week was." After everyone shares, you could use your facilitating, linking, and initiating skills (see page 29) to find a couple of common threads to expand on to generate some discussion. Or, be creative. Based on what you've learned about the group members thus far, come up with your own meaningful check-in activity. Limit check-in to about 15 minutes.

Education

Before the meeting, read through the *Workbook*'s Lesson Three in its entirety and pick two topics and two accompanying questions to explore during today's meeting. The major topics are the brain lobes, the cognitive functions, cognitive-function testing, activities of daily living, the stages of dementia, and dementia medications. The two I tend to select are cognitive function (because it also involves understanding the brain lobes) and stages of dementia (because cognitive-function test results and activities of daily living are part of the staging system, and questions about medications often come up when discussing stages).

Read aloud about the five cognitive functions (attention and concentration, memory and learning, executive function, language, and visuospatial function) and three related brain functions (personality, mood, and orientation) starting on page 76 of Lesson Three continuing to the top of page 79. Have group members follow along in their own copies of the *Workbook* as you read.

If you want to take a couple of extra minutes on this topic, ask one of the group members to then read aloud the story of Stephanie and Ray on pages 63 to 64. This is a good story to reinforce the importance of memory, which is one of the main functions of the temporal lobe, and bring up the topic of repetitive questions, one of the most common (and challenging) symptoms of Alzheimer's disease.

Then move ahead to pages 84 to 88, which describe the stages of dementia. Appendix 8 lists the instrumental and basic activities of daily living and the dementia stages, which you can provide to group members for the first discussion question. It will take 20 to 30 minutes to provide the educational information for this week's meeting.

As an aside, many care partners have questions about the medications used to treat people with dementia. If this is the case for your group, you could consider adding an extra meeting and invite a dementia specialist in to talk about this topic—a neurologist, geriatrician, psychiatrist, or advanced-practice practitioner like a physician assistant or nurse practitioner who specializes in diagnosing and treating dementia. Care partners (and leaders) find a medication-focused meeting to be interesting, educational, and valuable in their loved one's care.

Discussion
The questions on the top of page 89 in the *Workbook* are the main discussion questions for this week. Have members go through the Appendix 8 worksheets, and check off the symptoms of dementia their

loved one has had and is currently experiencing. Then ask: "Based on the descriptions of the stages of dementia and what you checked on your worksheet, which stage would you say your loved one is in? How do you feel about this?" Then try, as best you can, to give everyone time to respond, realizing this may mean members only have about five minutes each, depending on the number you have.

Members may express sadness, worry, anxiety, and discouragement as they realize their loved one's stage is further along than they thought. Or, they may have similar emotions for a different reason—the life expectancy for someone with Alzheimer's disease, for example, is eight to ten years, and if their loved one is only in the early stage, they may be realizing that their caregiving responsibilities will last for years and years more.

If you have time to discuss a second question, I would suggest the question on cognitive function from pages 77 to 78: "Now that you've learned about the cognitive functions, please describe any dementia symptoms your loved one may be having related to attention and concentration, memory and learning, executive function, language, and visuospatial function." Ask members to pick one cognitive function that's affected in their loved one, and what the associated symptom is.

Preview and closing

If you have time and want to have an end-of-meeting Mindfulness Moment, please do so. Otherwise, tell the group members you will be transitioning to a completely new topic next week—Lesson Four: Adapting to Changing Relationships. You'll be talking about a number of common behavior changes that are caused by dementia, the impact these behaviors have on relationships, and ways to adapt. Adapting to changing relationships is Central Need 3 of dementia care partners. Wish everyone well, then dismiss the group. Three meetings down, seven to go!

MEETING FOUR
ADAPTING TO CHANGING RELATIONSHIPS

Note: Review the Appendix 4 overview and the previous section "Anatomy of a meeting plan" for information relevant to all meetings.

Meeting overview and key topics

Lesson Four revolves around the theme of changing relationships between the person with dementia and their care partner due to the effects of the dementia on brain function, including cognitive function, personality, mood, and orientation. The meeting is organized into three areas: attachment and attachment loss, behavior changes and relationship challenges in early- and middle-stage dementia, and ways to adapt to those changes, which is Central Need 3 of dementia care partners. The educational topics reflect these three areas, whereas the discussion questions will focus on the behavior changes their loved ones are experiencing and how they affect relationships, as well as ways to adapt, emphasizing a very easy-to-remember and helpful strategy that I refer to as AAR—acknowledge, affirm, and redirect. By this point in the group's development, you should be past the forming and hopefully the storming stages so that the norming can begin.

Opening and Mindfulness Moment

Open with a brief "welcome" and move into the Mindfulness Moment. Then go straight to the breathing exercise without reading the description of what mindfulness is.

Check-in

For check-in, you have a couple of options. You may prefer the quicker check-in I described for last week's meeting ("Let's take time for a quick check-in. Who from the group would like to share a particular success or challenge from the past week?") Or you could ask members if they have questions or reflections about the last two weeks of educational content—what dementia is, the different types of dementia, the brain lobes and their function, cognitive function, instrumental and basic activities of daily living, and the stages of dementia. I find the education from Lessons Two and Three on these topics helps care partners understand why their loved one does the challenging things they do (e.g., repetitive questions), or why they can't do certain things (e.g., remember, multitask, and get words out). Don't feel as though you need to be a brain expert to answer questions that arise. What's most important is that the care partner is given the freedom to ask their questions in a safe space. You can always report back next week on an answer you had to look up, or suggest the care partner ask the question of their loved one's medical provider.

Education

As mentioned, the educational component of this meeting will cover three things: attachment, behavior changes, and adaptations. Attachment theory, attachment loss, and separation distress are described on pages 98 to 100 of *The Dementia Care-Partner's Workbook*. You can read these pages out loud to group members, or provide a synopsis of the main concepts: attachment, secure versus insecure attachment, and separation-distress behaviors (seeking and withdrawal responses). Pages 101 through 116 describe the many different behavior changes and relationship challenges that occur in early- to middle-stage dementia, for the most part regardless of dementia type.

Because you cannot feasibly cover all this material, provide brief definitions of a subset of your choosing (perhaps behaviors being expressed by the loved ones of group members), or you can use this list: apathy, loss of insight/denial, emotional withdrawal/loss of empathy, depression/anxiety, repetitive questions/vocalizations, lost identity, paranoid delusions, and behavioral disinhibition. Members will identify with one or several of these, which they'll have a chance to discuss shortly.

Finally, mention that the *Workbook* provides five strategies to adapt to these behavior changes, on pages 116 to 130. You can describe the first two briefly, patience (page 117) and acknowledge-affirm-redirect (AAR, pages 117 to 118), leaving the others for members to read about on their own. The five love languages (pages 120 to 128) is a strategy that was the topic of a prior book I co-authored: *Keeping Love Alive as Memories Fade: The 5 Love Languages and the Alzheimer's Journey.* You could consider adding an extra meeting to cover this topic.

Discussion

Because behavior changes and relationship challenges are so common, you are likely to have ample discussion without much prompting. This is also a topic where members can share their own experience with others who have experienced similar changes/challenges. For the first discussion question, read the list of the behaviors you just discussed— apathy, loss of insight/denial, emotional withdrawal/loss of empathy, depression/anxiety, repetitive questions/vocalizations, lost identity, paranoid delusions, and behavioral disinhibition—then use this prompt: "Describe the one behavior your loved one has experienced that has been the most challenging for you and your relationship with them."

Encourage members to share similar experiences by saying something like: "Has anyone else in the group experienced what Ann is describing?" Join people with like experiences by using your counseling skills, such as facilitating, linking, and initiating. Reinforce concepts of attachment theory, attachment loss, and separation distress when appropriate.

This is where the group should evolve to the third phase (the norming stage), characterized by in-depth self-exploration and encountering the pain of caregiving. And while you will certainly be a comforting presence to them, hopefully care partners with similar experiences will begin lasting friendships as co-journeyers.

If there is time for a second discussion topic/question, briefly define the AAR strategy again, then read the story about the man who had the delusion of his wife's infidelity, on pages 118 to 119. Now ask members if there is a behavior challenge they've experienced that might benefit from AAR. Help them talk through how they would acknowledge, affirm, and redirect. Let other group members join in the discussion voluntarily, or ask members who did not get a chance to share during the first discussion question about their thoughts. Encourage members who are using AAR and other strategies for managing challenging behaviors successfully, and acknowledge how hard this aspect of a loved one's care is for care partners who are struggling. You will probably run out of time before accomplishing what you'd hoped for this meeting, but that's OK—it's about the group's agenda and needs, not yours!

Preview and closing

If you have time and want to have an end-of-meeting Mindfulness Moment, please do so. Otherwise, tell the group members you will be transitioning to a completely new topic next week— Lesson Five: Coping with Grief and Loss. You'll learn about the nature of grief, which is what you think and feel on the inside in response to loss, and mourning, the outward expression of your grief, and why they are both necessary parts of the caregiving journey that address Central Need 4— Grieve your losses. Wish everyone well, then dismiss the group. Four meetings down, six to go!

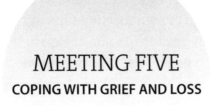

MEETING FIVE
COPING WITH GRIEF AND LOSS

Note: Review the Appendix 4 overview and the previous section "Anatomy of a meeting plan" for information relevant to all meetings.

Meeting overview and key topics

Lesson Five, which focuses on the grief and loss associated with being a dementia care partner, naturally follows Lesson Four since much of the grief is related to relationship changes. Members will readily identify with the content of this meeting, and will continue to self-explore and experience the pain of their losses. The meeting has three related content areas that will be the focus of both the education and discussion components—the definitions of grief and mourning, the kinds of losses dementia care partners experience (personal, relationship, peace of mind), and family grief and loss. By now you should have a good sense of how much time you want to devote to check-in, education, and discussion, so plan your time accordingly for this meeting.

Opening and Mindfulness Moment

Open with a brief "welcome" and move into the Mindfulness Moment. Then go straight to the breathing exercise without reading the description of what mindfulness is.

Check-in

For check-in, again decide between a quick check-in or a longer one, perhaps asking group members to reflect on last week's meeting on behavior changes, relationship challenges, and the AAR strategy. Or, if you want to try something a bit different, try this question: "We're at the halfway point in our ten-meeting support group. Has the group been helpful, or has it unearthed some unexpected challenges for you?" By now you are likely getting a sense of what your group needs as far as check-in is concerned.

Education

As mentioned, the education will include three topics—the definitions of grief and mourning, the kinds of losses dementia care partners experience, and family grief and loss. If check-in was on the longer side, you could omit the third topic.

The difference between grief and mourning, one of the most important teachings of the *Leader's Manual's* co-author Dr. Alan Wolfelt (I wholeheartedly recommend his amazing book *Understanding Your Grief*), is extremely important for members to understand. The definition of grief is on page 135, and mourning is on page 136, of Lesson Five, which you can read aloud to the group. Emphasize this important notion: "While grief usually comes naturally, you will have to make an intentional effort to mourn. That's why telling your story is the first central need of dementia care partners. It's an act of mourning essential to your well-being."

Next you'll discuss the personal losses, relationship losses, and loss of peace of mind that care partners experience. Summarize the content from pages 138 to 144 of *The Dementia Care-Partner's Workbook*. You can have members take turns reading the bullets on pages 139 and 141. These losses are often associated with deep pain. Be prepared for heartfelt expressions of mourning to occur in the discussion that follows. If you decide to mention family grief and loss, read the paragraph that starts at the bottom of page 146 ("In a typical family ...) and finishes at the top of the following page. This will provide sufficient background for the discussion question on family conflict.

Discussion

Just like last meeting's discussion on behavior changes and relationship challenges, this lesson's discussion should need little prompting before the group "takes off and runs!" Here are some questions to consider asking, in no particular order. You may only have time for one question, so choose that which best fits your group.

- "Describe the feelings of grief you're experiencing as care partner to your loved one with Alzheimer's disease or whatever type of dementia they have. How have you mourned (outwardly expressed your feelings of grief)?"

- "What sorts of losses have you experienced as a dementia care partner—time for yourself, family and friends, your own medical and mental health, your job/career, relational intimacy, plans for the future, and/or peace of mind?"

- "Has your family experienced conflict as a consequence of your loved one's dementia journey? Please describe this for the group."

You will probably again run out of time before accomplishing what you'd planned for this meeting, but that's part of letting the group do what it needs to do, and at this point, the group is norming, getting ready to enter the important working stage.

Preview and closing

If you have time and want to have an end-of-meeting Mindfulness Moment, please do so. Otherwise, let group members know you will be transitioning to yet another new topic next week—Lesson Six: Stress and Self-Care, which addresses Central Need 5—Take care of yourself and Central Need 6—Ask for and accept help from others. Taking care of themselves and getting help are two things most dementia care partners do not do a very good job of. For those who like to read ahead, point them to the Wellness Wheel on page 164 of Lesson Six. You'll have an activity around this next week. Wish everyone well, then dismiss the group. Five meetings down, five to go!

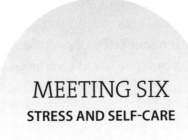

MEETING SIX
STRESS AND SELF-CARE

Note: Review the Appendix 4 overview and the previous section "Anatomy of a meeting plan" for information relevant to all meetings.

Meeting overview and key topics

The content of Lesson Six is divided between common reactions dementia care partners have to the many challenges of caregiving, such as depression, anxiety, and stress, and its impact on physical, emotional, and spiritual health, and care-partner wellness, an ideal state of being that would occur if it was possible to meet everyone's needs in a balanced way. Of the eight central needs of dementia care partners, the two that seem the hardest to address and meet are Central Need 5 — Take care of yourself and Central Need 6 — Ask for and accept help from others, which are obviously interrelated. In this meeting, a transition will occur in the group's progress. The education and discussion around the topic of wellness will move group members and the group as a whole into the fourth phase, which is the commitment to healing and growth, also known as the working stage. Are you ready? Let's do it!

Opening and Mindfulness Moment

Open with a brief "welcome" and move into the Mindfulness Moment. Then go straight to the breathing exercise without reading the description of what mindfulness is.

Check-in

For check-in, once again you can decide between a quick check-in, asking members how that last week was, or a longer one, asking group members to reflect on last week's meeting on grief and loss, something along the lines of: "Think about last week's discussion on the grief and losses you experience as care partner to your loved one with dementia. How are you grieving? In other words, what feelings do you have on the inside? How are you mourning? How have you outwardly expressed your grief? Through reading Lesson Five or from the group meeting on grief and loss, what new insights do you have on the inevitable losses that occur on the dementia journey?" Any one of these questions should stimulate a good discussion for check-in. For the remaining four check-ins, the emphasis will be on healing, growth, and resilience.

Education

The educational aspects of Lesson Six lend themselves to group participation, so begin by having everyone open their copy of *The Dementia Care-Partner's Workbook* to page 154. You can then read aloud the introductory paragraph ("Of all the personal challenges ...") and have members read the nine symptoms of depression on pages 154 to 155, then the six symptoms of anxiety on pages 157 to 158.

Now take a moment to summarize the text surrounding these symptom lists, specifically differentiating between sadness versus depression and concern versus anxiety. Then read aloud the introductory paragraph about stress on the top of page 160, and have members again take turns reading the eleven symptoms of stress. You can briefly discuss the difference between acute and chronic stress, and mention that chronic stress can have effects on physical and mental health as well as physical appearance.

The education about wellness will be integrated into the Wellness Wheel activity, which I'll describe in the discussion section below. Finish the educational component of the lesson by reading aloud page 176 of the *Workbook* on assembling a team, ending with, "... receive the grace others extend to you."

Discussion

Try to plan out the Lesson Six meeting so you have time for two discussion questions. Spend less time on the first question, more on the second one. Dementia care partners are a stressed lot, so getting them to talk about their stress won't be difficult. Have them turn to pages 151 to 152 of *The Dementia Care-Partner's Workbook* and read through the Alzheimer's Association's ten symptoms of caregiver stress, selecting the one symptom that best describes them right now. This list includes symptoms of depression, anxiety, and physical, mental, and spiritual stress. Then have each member spend a couple of minutes describing why that one symptom fits them. This question is a good lead-in to some education and discussion about wellness.

Go ahead and hand out the Wellness Wheel, which is Appendix 9 of the *Leader's Manual*. Then turn to page 163 in the *Workbook* and read the definition of wellness, starting with, "What exactly is wellness?" Members will be able to see the eight components of wellness on their Wellness Wheel. Allow a few minutes for everyone to read the definitions of the four components on the left half of the page—physical, emotional, social, and spiritual. Ask them to choose one of these four and make a goal for that component that will promote self-care and wellness. For example, a goal to improve physical health might be making the time to get a massage once a month. Then have each member spend a couple of minutes sharing their wellness goal.

After everyone has shared, point them to pages 175 to 176 in the *Workbook*, which has instructions for them to create their own personal wellness plan (it's also provided as the second page of Appendix 9). They're one-quarter of the way to having a wellness plan, having already chosen a goal in one area of wellness. You could ask members to complete their wellness plan over the next week and bring it to class next meeting to share with the group during check-in.

Preview and closing

If you have time and want to have an end-of-meeting Mindfulness

Moment, please do so. Otherwise, let group members know about plans for next week's meeting, which is Lesson Seven: Getting More Help and Transitioning Care—a logical extension of this meeting. It explores options for additional help when dementia has progressed to the point that more help is needed. Help from a home-health agency, as well as the difficult topic of transitioning care to a residential setting, like assisted living, memory care, or a nursing home, are discussed. Lesson Seven, like the prior lesson, also focuses on Central Need 6—Ask for and accept help from others, as well as Central Need 7—Prepare for what's ahead. Wish everyone well, then dismiss the group. Six meetings down, four to go!

MEETING SEVEN
GETTING MORE HELP AND TRANSITIONING CARE

Note: Review the Appendix 4 overview and the previous section "Anatomy of a meeting plan" for information relevant to all meetings.

Meeting overview and key topics

Lesson Seven describes options for additional help in middle- and late-stage dementia, such as a certified nursing assistant from a home-health agency coming into the home or the transition of care to a residential setting, like assisted living, memory care, or a nursing home. The need for more help is usually triggered by one of the behavior changes that occurs with later-stage dementia, such as agitation and aggression, hallucinations, wandering, sexual behaviors, resisting or refusing care, sundowning, day-night reversal, and incontinence. The overarching purpose of Lesson Seven is to motivate care partners to get the help they need when the going gets really tough, which it does in the latter part of the middle stage and the late stage, when these hard-to-handle behaviors occur. Accepting that more help is needed, then actually getting that help, is a big step that not only improves care for the loved one with dementia, it helps the care partner exercise better self-care.

Opening and Mindfulness Moment

Open with a brief "welcome" and move into the Mindfulness Moment. Then go straight to the breathing exercise without reading the description of what mindfulness is.

Check-in

For this week's check-in, have members pull from their wellness plan on page 176 of *The Dementia Care-Partner's Workbook*. Ask them to share some of their wellness goals. You can do this in a couple of different ways. One option is to have individuals describe their goals for physical, emotional, social, and spiritual wellness, or you could ask the group: "Would some of you be willing to share your goals for spiritual wellness?" You can even share with everyone that they've entered the fourth phase of group growth, known as the working stage, in which they are to make a commitment to their own healing and growth, a necessity given the reality of the stress associated with being a dementia care partner. Congratulate them on setting wellness goals— and maybe even pass around pieces of dark chocolate to celebrate!

Education

Once again, there is a lot of educational material in the lesson, more than can be covered in 90 minutes, so you'll need to be selective about what you present and let members supplement that with their own reading.

Begin by reading the first line of Lesson Seven in the *Workbook*: "I hope the last meeting on self-care and wellness convinced you that caregiving is a team sport. We will carry this important thought into the present meeting and add that **dementia caregiving is a marathon, not a sprint**." Then read the paragraph that starts on the bottom of page 179 ("In Lesson Four ...") and continues to the top of page 180 (ends with, " ... loved one at home"). This is a good lead into the challenging behaviors of later-stage dementia, which are described on pages 182 to 195. Briefly summarize each of them in a sentence or two, including agitation and aggression, hallucinations, wandering, sexual behaviors, resisting or refusing care, sundowning, day-night reversal, and incontinence.

In keeping with the theme of the group being in the working stage, introduce the options for getting more help as having a two-fold purpose: helping their loved one get the best possible care given where they are in their dementia journey, and helping them as care partner continue their own commitment to personal healing and wellness. Of all the options for getting more help, the three most often used are home-health agencies, adult daycare, and memory-care facilities. These are discussed on pages 198 to 200 and 204 to 205 of the *Workbook*, which you can summarize for your group members.

A couple of other resources you might want to mention, if you have them in your community, are the Area Agencies on Aging (page 198) and the PACE program (page 207). Lastly, if you have a significant number of group members who have a loved one in residential care, whether it be assisted living, memory care, or a nursing home, you might want to have the group read through the "Helpful Hints" on pages 209 to 210.

Discussion

For this meeting, one discussion question usually is enough to fill the entire discussion time. The question is: "Describe a behavioral challenge or situation in which you have thought, 'I don't know if I can manage by myself any longer' or 'I don't know if I can manage him (or her) at home any longer.'" While this meeting's discussion will elicit some of the most difficult caregiving situations care partners experience, resist the temptation to provide quick advice or solutions. Rather, use your counseling skills to help members acknowledge the challenges of their particular situation, understand why their loved one is behaving as they are, and explore the possibilities they have to meet their loved one's needs while keeping their own wellness in mind. Skills such as reflecting feelings (these are often very emotional scenarios), restating, clarifying, evaluating, and giving feedback are some of the skills that may be most helpful. For example: "Janet, I hear you describing some real challenges getting your mom to take a shower, even once a week. She seems to be actively resisting your care. This must be very frustrating for you. Sometimes a parent does not want their adult child to help them meet basic personal-care needs—it's a dignity issue. Have you thought about a paid caregiver to come in a couple of times a week to help mom shower and give you a break for some self-care? What do others in the group think?" By responding in this way, you've empathized with Janet's situation, helped her think through a difficult situation utilizing a "win-win" approach, and drawn on the group's experience to help her.

Preview and closing

If you have time and want to have an end-of-meeting Mindfulness Moment, please do so. Otherwise, tell the group members you will be transitioning to an important and related group of topics in Lesson Eight: Legal, Financial, and End-of-Life Issues. Like the last couple of meetings, this one will also help address Central Need 7—Prepare for what's ahead. Wish everyone well, then dismiss the group. Seven meetings down, three to go!

MEETING EIGHT
LEGAL, FINANCIAL, AND END-OF-LIFE ISSUES

Note: Review the Appendix 4 overview and the previous section "Anatomy of a meeting plan" for information relevant to all meetings.

Meeting overview and key topics

This meeting encompasses a range of issues in three related areas—legal, financial, and end-of-life. In our dementia care-partner support groups at Wake Forest Baptist Health, we always have one of the local elder-law attorneys come for at least part of the meeting, and members find this one of the most practical and useful meetings in the entire curriculum, simply because they tend to be in a more reactive than proactive mode given all they have to do and the paucity of time to do it in. Therefore, Lesson Eight serves more of a utilitarian function. There are simply certain things every person with dementia and their family (and in reality, any of us entering the senior years of our lives) must have in place—legally, financially, and for the end-of-life—to make a difficulty journey as hiccup-free as possible.

Opening and Mindfulness Moment

Open with a brief "welcome" and move into the Mindfulness Moment. Then go straight to the breathing exercise without reading the description of what mindfulness is.

Check-in

If you have an elder-law attorney coming as a guest speaker for this week, and they come for the start of the meeting, have group members introduce themselves, provide their loved one's name and what their diagnosis is, and what stage they are in (mild cognitive impairment, early-, middle-, or late-stage dementia). If you are not having an elder-law attorney come, or they aren't coming until after check-in, ask group members to share their thoughts and feelings about the last meeting on the behavior challenges of later-stage dementia and getting more help. By now members should be looking more at one another during check-in rather than just at you. Encourage this with your facilitating, linking, and initiating skills.

Education

For education, if you have an elder-law attorney, you can provide the attorney with a copy of Lesson Eight from *The Dementia Care-Partner's Workbook*, or they may prefer to use a handout of their own. If you will be providing the education, you can divide the education time into thirds, covering selected legal, financial, and end-of-life topics.

First, provide members brief descriptions of the durable power of attorney and healthcare power of attorney (pages 218 to 219). All members will likely have at least heard of the Health Insurance Portability and Accountability Act (HIPAA), but they may not be aware that they as care partners need to be listed on their loved one's HIPAA form so they can freely communicate with the doctor and other medical and mental-health providers.

If driving issues are relevant to any members of the group, you can read the middle paragraph on page 224 ("But driving is ...") to provide information on why driving is such a complex task, then defer questions on driving to the discussion time.

Next, give brief descriptions of wills and trusts (page 227 to 228). You can refer group members to review the examples of the Smiths and Millers on their own (pages 229 to 232) as a way to learn about the cost of care.

Last, briefly describe the living will, do not resuscitate, and physician's orders for life-sustaining treatment documents (pages 240 to 241), as well as selected end-of-life issues (fluids, feeding, CPR/respirator, antibiotics, and hip fracture) on pages 236 to 238.

Discussion

The discussion time will be taken up by questions for the elder-law attorney if you have one coming. Otherwise, the following questions allow members to articulate what's most on their mind and heart across this broad range of interrelated issues. They are: "Based on everything covered in the meeting, what is the one thing in the areas of legal, financial, and end-of-life issues related to your loved one's dementia journey you feel the least prepared for? What would you need to do in order to be more prepared for this?"

You could also talk specifically about end-of-life issues with this question: "Have you discussed some of the end-of-life decisions with your loved one or as a family? Which one is the most challenging for you to consider, and why?" These questions lend themselves well to group discussion. As you did with check-in, encourage members to respond to and support one another by using facilitating, linking, and initiating skills.

Preview and closing

If you have time and want to have an end-of-meeting Mindfulness Moment, please do so. Otherwise, tell the group members you will be transitioning to a very different topic that is thought-provoking, challenging, and contemplative all at the same time—Lesson Nine: Existential and Spiritual Questions, which addresses Central Need 8—Explore existential and spiritual questions to find meaning. These questions of faith naturally come up when bad things happen to good people. Wish everyone well, then dismiss the group. Eight meetings down, two to go!

MEETING NINE
EXISTENTIAL AND SPIRITUAL QUESTIONS

Note: Review the Appendix 4 overview and the previous section "Anatomy of a meeting plan" for information relevant to all meetings.

Meeting overview and key topics

Lesson Nine on existential and spiritual questions is positioned near the end of the curriculum on purpose. Members will be challenged by this topic on an individual level, and the group will be challenged as a whole, since these questions are not necessarily ones that have answers. What's most important is being able to ask them, and at this point in the group's development, members are familiar, comfortable, and trusting with one another, which allows them to feel safe in their vulnerability. As leader, this may be the meeting in which you speak the least, but it will be important for you to be "on your toes" since the discussion of existential and spiritual issues can bring out Holly (the holy roller) and Paul (the preacher). Brush up on your evaluating, giving feedback, blocking, and protecting skills as these may be necessary if religiosity or advice-giving dominates the conversation!

Opening and Mindfulness Moment

Open with a brief "welcome" and move into the Mindfulness Moment. Then go straight to the breathing exercise without reading the description of what mindfulness is.

Check-in

This week's check-in should focus on members' thoughts, feelings, and questions in response to last week's meeting on legal, financial, and end-of-life issues. Consider letting one of the members decide what the check-in should be about by asking: "I wonder if one of you has a question or issue they would like to get the group's input on? If so, please feel free to lead our check-in time for us." You could also ask someone in the group to do this ahead of time if there is a member you feel is up to the task.

Education

Begin the education portion of the meeting by reading the introduction to Lesson Nine in *The Dementia Care Partner* Workbook (page 245 to the top of 246) as well as the section entitled "Why Ask Why" (page 251 to the top of 252). You can also summarize Viktor Frankl's life story and the ways in which he suggests meaning can be found even in the most challenging of circumstances, from pages 252 to 259 , if you would like to provide this additional educational content.

Discussion

For discussion, the group will need little prompting to have a vigorous, engaging interchange. You can review the various journaling prompts in the *Workbook's* Lesson Nine and choose one or two questions to ask, or you can pick from the ones I've selected for you below. They are:

- Has your loved one's dementia journey challenged or strengthened your faith or spirituality? Please share your thoughts about this with the group.

- The end of the lesson has six existential and spiritually focused quotes from six very different people. Select the one that speaks the most to you, and share why.

"I am learning to trust the journey even when I do not understand it."
— Mila Bron

"Trust that everything happens for a reason, even when you're not wise enough to understand it."
— Oprah Winfrey

"Someday you will look back and understand why it happened the way it did."
— Boniface Z. Zulu

"Sometimes...bad things happen to inspire you to change and grow."
— Robert Tew

"When something bad happens, you have three choices. You can either let it define you, let it destroy you, or you can let it strengthen you."
— Dr. Seuss

"Sometimes what we think is a setback is really a setup for God to do something great."
— Joel Osteen

Preview and closing

If you have time and want to have an end-of-meeting Mindfulness Moment, please do so. Otherwise, tell the group members that next week is the last meeting together, and it will cover Lesson Ten: Retelling Your Story Starting Today (Central Need One). Encourage them to complete the journaling questions in Lesson Ten regarding Central Needs Two through Eight, which will be the focus of next week's final check-in/discussion.

MEETING TEN

RETELLING YOUR STORY STARTING TODAY

Note: Review the Appendix 4 overview and the previous section "Anatomy of a meeting plan" for information relevant to all meetings.

Meeting overview and key topics

In preparation for this final group meeting, review the information on Phase Five: Preparation for and leaving the group (the closing stage) from pages 40 to 42 of *A Leader's Manual*. Encourage members to think of today or tonight as their graduation, celebrating their accomplishment of working through all the content in the ten lessons of *The Dementia Care-Partner's Workbook*, the forging of new friendships, learning new skills and ways to cope, and being aware of the need for self-care and wellness.

Opening and Mindfulness Moment

If you had members complete baseline assessments in the first week, you can hand them the same assessments when they arrive and ask them to complete and turn them in to you before group starts. This is also a good time to have them complete the Support-Group Participant Evaluation Form (Appendix 10). When ready, open with an acknowledgment that this is the last meeting, and as such, this will be the last Mindfulness Moment the group will do together. Encourage members to continue daily mindfulness practices, and point them to the mindfulness books and apps in the Resources section at the back of the *Workbook*.

Check-in, education, and discussion

The check-in, education, and discussion components of the last meeting will occur together for the last lesson. Read the "Looking Back" content on page 267 of Lesson Ten (you can have group members alternate reading the eight central needs). Then ask this question for the group to discuss: "Pick the one central need out of the eight that you feel you've made the most progress toward addressing over the last ten weeks. Share what you have learned with the group." And if there is time, have members share the one central need they made the least progress in addressing, and why this particular one has been so challenging for them.

Yarn toss

The yarn toss is my favorite closing activity of all. It is simple to do. Give one member of the group a ball of yarn. As them to loop a piece around one of their fingers, then answer this question: "Describe what this ten-week support group experience has been like for you. Feel free to share how it has helped, how it has challenged you, and who or what you'll remember most from the group. Then toss the ball of yarn across the circle to another group member." After all the members have shared, then you and your co-leader(s) should take turns telling the group what they have meant to you. One of my work colleagues likes to name a "gift" that either a member of the group (or the group itself) has given her. For example: "I feel like Janet gave me a gift throughout this group because she consistently demonstrated vulnerability. This is something that has always been difficult for me. Janet, your willingness to be vulnerable has truly been an encouragement to me. Thank you for that." This may trigger group members to share how others in the group, or the leaders, have gifted them. When everyone has spoken, take a scissors and cut the string down the middle of the web of yarn in such a way that everyone has a piece to take home with them as a way to remember the group experience.

Resources

In the last meeting, I like to provide members with a resource packet to take with them. If you are planning to have monthly maintenance dementia care-partner support groups, provide a flyer that gives information on when and where the group will meet and who will be leading it. Hand out the Resource List (Appendix 11), which has a listing of helpful books, websites, and the like. Other information you can provide might include brochures or pamphlets on local adult daycare programs, Area Agency on Aging, PACE program, residential-care facilities, continuing-care retirement communities, elder-law attorneys, geriatric case managers—the list could go on and on. You can also pass out the list with names and contact information for members who agreed to share this information at the first week's sign-in.

Closing

Having provided the resources, you can now bring the meeting to a close, wishing everyone well. Distribute the Certificate of Dementia Care-Partner Support Group Participation (Appendix 12). Anticipate members will linger as they say their goodbyes. Congratulations on a job well done!

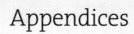

Appendices

Appendix 1: Support Group Ground Rules...........................107

Appendix 2: Zarit Caregiver Burden Scale...........................109

Appendix 3: Geriatric Depression Scale and
Geriatric Anxiety Scale...113

Appendix 4: Support Group Leader's Overview......................117

Appendix 5: The Eight Central Needs of
Dementia Care Partners..127

Appendix 6: Symptoms of the Four Most
Common Forms of Dementia 129

Appendix 7: Understanding Our Emotions Exercise.................133

Appendix 8: Activities of Daily Living and
the Stages of Dementia...135

Appendix 9: Wellness Wheel and Wellness Plan....................141

Appendix 10: Support-Group Participant Evaluation Form..........145

Appendix 11: Resource for Support Group Members 151

Appendix 12: Certificate of Dementia Care-Partner
Support Group Participation 155

Support Group
Ground Rules

APPENDIX 1

We welcome you to our support group. We understand the courage and strength it takes to attend a support group like this. The purpose of the support group is to provide education, understanding, and hope to care partners who have a loved one with dementia. Our hope is that the group will be a safe place for you to come and meet others who are on a similar journey as you. At right are the ground rules we will follow during our meetings.

SUPPORT GROUP GROUND RULES

1. **We recognize and respect our differences.** We recognize that everyone's journey is unique to them. We respect and offer compassion to all members, even if their experiences, beliefs, and views are different than our own.

2. **We acknowledge that there is no quick fix or set timetable** for becoming reconciled to or accepting that our loved one has dementia. We will be patient with one another as we process our thoughts and emotions over time.

3. **We encourage all group members to speak freely,** as it helps build support, encouragement, and understanding among group members. We also recognize that sometimes we may prefer to listen rather than speak.

4. **We are compassionate listeners.** We agree that only one person will speak at a time, without interruption. We will give each group member the time they need to share. We listen without judgment or criticism and offer each other acceptance.

5. **We speak only about ourselves and our experience**, using "I" or "we" statements to discuss what has been helpful to us. We will not give advice to others unless asked.

6. **We respect the privacy of each group member**. We agree not to discuss any information about other members outside of the group, though we do encourage group members to spend time with one another during and after the weeks our group meets. The group leaders will respect the privacy of members except in the following circumstances: 1) members who are thought to be suicidal; 2) members who threaten to harm another; 3) child or elder abuse is suspected; or 4) legal subpoenas.

7. **We agree to attend each meeting and be on time.** If we know we will be absent on a given week, we will let one of the leaders know.

8. **We agree to be mentally present for each meeting**. We agree to attend group meetings "clean and sober." If we are struggling with drugs or alcohol, we will let a leader know so we can receive help.

Please keep these ground rules with you and refer to them from time to time to keep them fresh in your mind. Thank you!

Zarit Caregiver Burden Scale

APPENDIX 2

Care Partner's Name: _____

Date:_____

The following questions reflect how people sometimes feel when they are taking care of another person. After each question, circle how often you feel that way: never, rarely, sometimes, frequently, or nearly always. There are no right or wrong answers.

	Never	Rarely	Sometimes	Frequently	Nearly always
1. Do you feel that your loved one asks for more help than he or she needs?	0	1	2	3	4
2. Do you feel that because of the time you spend with your loved one, you do not have enough time for yourself?	0	1	2	3	4
3. Do you feel stress between caring for your loved one and trying to meet other responsibilities for your family or work?	0	1	2	3	4

	Never	Rarely	Sometimes	Frequently	Nearly always
4. Do you feel embarrassed over your loved one's behavior?	0	1	2	3	4
5. Do you feel angry when you are around your loved one?	0	1	2	3	4
6. Do you feel that your loved one currently affects your relationship with other family members or friends in a negative way?	0	1	2	3	4
7. Are you afraid about what the future holds for your loved one?	0	1	2	3	4
8. Do you feel your loved one is dependent on you?	0	1	2	3	4
9. Do you feel strained when you are around your loved one?	0	1	2	3	4
10. Do you feel your health has suffered because of your involvement with your loved one?	0	1	2	3	4
11. Do you feel that you do not have as much privacy as you would like, because of your loved one?	0	1	2	3	4
12. Do you feel that your social life has suffered because you are caring for your loved one?	0	1	2	3	4
13. Do you feel uncomfortable about having friends over, because of your loved one?	0	1	2	3	4
14. Do you feel that your loved one seems to expect you to take care of him or her, as if you were the only one he or she could depend on?	0	1	2	3	4
15. Do you feel that you do not have enough money to care for your loved one, in addition to the rest of your expenses?	0	1	2	3	4
16. Do you feel that you will be unable to take care of your loved one much longer?	0	1	2	3	4

A Leader's Manual for Dementia Care-Partner Support Groups

	Never	Rarely	Sometimes	Frequently	Nearly always
17. Do you feel that you have lost control of your life since your loved one's illness?	0	1	2	3	4
18. Do you wish you could just leave the care of your loved one to someone else?	0	1	2	3	4
19. Do you feel uncertain about what to do about your loved one?	0	1	2	3	4
20. Do you feel you should be doing more for your loved one?	0	1	2	3	4
21. Do you feel you could be doing a better job in caring for your loved one?	0	1	2	3	4

	None	Little	Mild	Moderate	Severe
22. Overall, how burdened do you feel caring for your loved one?	0	1	2	3	4

Geriatric Anxiety Scale

APPENDIX 3

Care Partner's Name: _____

Date:_____

ANXIETY SCALE (SHORT VERSION)

Choose the best answer for how you have felt over the past WEEK:

1.	Do you feel nervous much of the time?	Yes	No
2.	Have you worried about your future this week?	Yes	No
3.	Do you feel that your life is too fast?	Yes	No
4.	Do you often get anxious?	Yes	No
5.	Have you felt relaxed most of today?	Yes	No
6.	Do you feel afraid at different times during the day?	Yes	No
7.	Do you feel stress-free most of the time?	Yes	No
8.	Does your stomach feel nervous much of the time?	Yes	No

9. Do you prefer to have someone with you most of the time?   Yes   No

10. Do you feel you have more anxiety than most?   Yes   No

11. Do you find it easy to sleep at night?   Yes   No

12. Do you feel pretty stressed now?   Yes   No

13. Do you feel you have more energy than yesterday?   Yes   No

14. Do you feel that you cannot remember things like you used to?   Yes   No

15. Do you think most people are less anxious than you?   Yes   No

Geriatric Depression Scale

APPENDIX 3

Care Partner's Name: _____

Date:_____

DEPRESSION SCALE (SHORT VERSION)

Choose the best answer for how you have felt over the past WEEK:

1. Are you basically satisfied with your life?   Yes   No

2. Have you dropped many of your activities
   and interests?   Yes   No

3. Do you feel that your life is empty?   Yes   No

4. Do you often get bored?   Yes   No

5. Are you in good spirits most of the time?   Yes   No

6. Are you afraid that something bad is
   going to happen to you?   Yes   No

7. Do you feel happy most of the time?   Yes   No

8. Do you often feel helpless?   Yes   No

9. Do you prefer to stay at home, rather than
    going out and doing new things?   Yes   No

10. Do you feel you have more problems with
    memory than most?   Yes   No

11. Do you think it is wonderful to be alive now?   Yes   No

12. Do you feel pretty worthless the way you are now?   Yes   No

13. Do you feel full of energy?   Yes   No

14. Do you feel that your situation is hopeless?   Yes   No

15. Do you think most people are better off than you?   Yes   No

Support Group Leader's Overview of Meetings

APPENDIX 4

1

MEETING WEEK: One

LESSON TITLE: Telling Your Story from the Beginning

LESSON OVERVIEW:
- Welcome members
- Leader intros
- Baseline assessments
- Review schedule
- Discuss journaling and homework
- Go over ground rules

EDUCATION AND DISCUSSION TOPICS:
- Eight central needs of dementia care partners
- Importance of telling your story

CENTRAL NEED(S) ADDRESSED:
- 1—Tell and retell your story

DISCUSSION QUESTIONS:
- What were your loved one's first symptoms of dementia?

HOMEWORK/OTHER:
- Distribute copies of *The Dementia Care-Partner's Workbook (TDCPW)*
- Read Lessons 1 and 2 *TDCPW*

2

MEETING WEEK: Two

LESSON TITLE: Basics of Alzheimer's Disease and Other Dementias

LESSON OVERVIEW: Understand what dementia is

EDUCATION AND DISCUSSION TOPICS:

- Dementia definition
- Symptoms of Alzheimer's, vascular, frontotemporal, and Lewy body dementia

CENTRAL NEED(S) ADDRESSED:

- 2—Educate yourself

DISCUSSION QUESTIONS:

- Understanding our emotions activity
- Q&A from Lessons 1 and 2 reading

HOMEWORK/OTHER:

- Read Lesson 3 *TDCPW*

THE EIGHT CENTRAL NEEDS OF DEMENTIA CARE PARTNERS ARE:

Central Need 1—Tell and retell your story

Central Need 2—Educate yourself

Central Need 3—Adapt to changing relationships

Central Need 4—Grieve your losses

Central Need 5—Take care of yourself

Central Need 6—Ask for and accept help from others

Central Need 7—Prepare for what's ahead

Central Need 8—Explore existential and spiritual questions to find meaning

3

MEETING WEEK: Three

LESSON TITLE:

Brain Structure and Function, Activities of Daily Living (ADL), and Dementia Stages

LESSON OVERVIEW:
- Understand functions of brain lobes
- Cognitive functions
- Instrumental and basic ADLs
- Dementia stages
- Meds

EDUCATION AND DISCUSSION TOPICS:
- Cognitive functions – attention, memory, executive, language, visuospatial
- Early-, middle-, and late-stage dementia

CENTRAL NEED(S) ADDRESSED:
- 2—Educate yourself

DISCUSSION QUESTIONS:
- Describe your loved one's dementia stage and cognitive symptoms

HOMEWORK/OTHER:
- Read Lesson 4 *TDCPW*

4

MEETING WEEK: Four

LESSON TITLE: Adapting to Changing Relationships

LESSON OVERVIEW:

Behavior changes in early- to middle-stage dementia and associated relationship challenges

EDUCATION AND DISCUSSION TOPICS:

- Behavior changes
- Ways to adapt – patience, AAR, KISSS, 5 love languages, and reminiscence approaches

CENTRAL NEED(S) ADDRESSED:

- 3—Adapt to changing relationships

DISCUSSION QUESTIONS:

- Behaviors loved one has - apathy, loss of insight/ denial, emotional withdrawal/loss of empathy, depression/anxiety, repetitive questions/ vocalizations, lost identity, paranoid delusions, and behavioral disinhibition
- Applying AAR strategy

HOMEWORK/OTHER:

- Read Lesson 5 *TDCPW*

5

MEETING WEEK: Five

LESSON TITLE: Coping with Grief and Loss

LESSON OVERVIEW:
- Grief vs mourning
- Kinds of losses
- Family grief

EDUCATION AND DISCUSSION TOPICS:
- Differences between grieving and mourning
- Personal losses, relationship losses, and loss of peace of mind

CENTRAL NEED(S) ADDRESSED:
- 4—Grieve your losses

DISCUSSION QUESTIONS:
- Care-partner grief and loss experiences
- Family conflict

HOMEWORK/OTHER:
- Read Lesson 6 *TDCPW*

6

MEETING WEEK: Six

LESSON TITLE: Stress and Self-Care

LESSON OVERVIEW:
- Care-partner depression, anxiety, stress
- Health and wellness

EDUCATION AND DISCUSSION TOPICS:
- Depression
- 6 symptoms of anxiety
- 11 symptoms of stress

CENTRAL NEED(S) ADDRESSED:
- 5—Take care of yourself
- 6—Ask for and accept help from others

DISCUSSION QUESTIONS:
- Describe symptoms of depression, anxiety, and stress
- Goals for mental, physical, social, and spiritual wellness

HOMEWORK/OTHER:
- Distribute Wellness Wheel and make Wellness Plan
- Read Lesson 7 *TDCPW*

7

LESSON TITLE: Getting More Help and Transitioning Care

LESSON OVERVIEW:
- Behaviors in middle- and late-stage dementia
- Home-health and residential-care options

EDUCATION AND DISCUSSION TOPICS:
- Describe behavior changes of later- stage dementia
- Home-health agencies, adult daycare, and memory-care residential-care facilities

CENTRAL NEED(S) ADDRESSED:
- 6—Ask for and accept help from others

DISCUSSION QUESTIONS:
- Describe loved one's symptoms: agitation and aggression, hallucinations, wandering, sexual behaviors, resisting or refusing care, sundowning, day-night reversal, and incontinence

HOMEWORK/OTHER:
- Read Lesson 8 *TDCPW*

8

MEETING WEEK: Eight

LESSON TITLE: Legal, Financial, and End-of-Life Issues

LESSON OVERVIEW: Plan ahead for legal, financial, and end-of-life issues

EDUCATION AND DISCUSSION TOPICS:
- Durable and healthcare POA, HIPAA, wills, trusts, living will,
  DNR, POLST documents
- End-of-life decisions

CENTRAL NEED(S) ADDRESSED:
- 7—Prepare for what's ahead

DISCUSSION QUESTIONS:
- Legal, financial, and end-of-life areas most/least prepared for
- Have end-of-life decisions been discussed?

HOMEWORK/OTHER:
- Read Lesson 9 *TDCPW*

A Leader's Manual for Dementia Care-Partner Support Groups

9

MEETING WEEK: Nine

LESSON TITLE: Existential and Spiritual Questions

LESSON OVERVIEW: Why me, why him/her questions

EDUCATION AND DISCUSSION TOPICS:
- Why ask why
- Frankl's philosophy of meaning of life

CENTRAL NEED(S) ADDRESSED:
- 8 — Explore existential and spiritual questions to find meaning

DISCUSSION QUESTIONS:
- Has journey challenged or strengthened faith?
- Spirituality quotes

HOMEWORK/OTHER:
- Read Lesson 10 *TDCPW*

10

LESSON TITLE: Retelling Your Story Starting Today

LESSON OVERVIEW:

- End-of-group assessments
- Group farewell

EDUCATION AND DISCUSSION TOPICS:

- Eight central needs of dementia care partners
- Importance of retelling story

CENTRAL NEED(S) ADDRESSED:

- 1 to 8

DISCUSSION QUESTIONS:

- Which central need has been best met?
- Which one still most challenging?

HOMEWORK/OTHER:

- Yarn toss activity
- Distribute end-of-group assessments, evaluation form, resources list, certificate of participation, and member contact information list.

The Eight Central Needs of Dementia Care Partners

APPENDIX 5

Central Need 1—Tell and retell your story
Being a dementia care partner is a stressful and often lonely, isolating experience. Telling and retelling your story, out loud to others and in writing, helps you vent about the demands and challenges of caregiving, clarify what you're thinking and feeling, and feel heard, less alone, and even validated.

Central Need 2—Educate yourself
Learning about Alzheimer's and the other forms of dementia, as well as the structure and function of the brain, and the many challenges of caregiving, will give you a better understanding of your loved one's symptoms and make you a more informed, empathetic, and effective care partner.

Central Need 3—Adapt to changing relationships
Dementia is a progressive disease that causes changes in your loved one's behavior, which in turn creates challenges in your relationship with them and others. These changes and challenges require you to adapt, and healthy adaptation allows you to stay meaningfully connected to your loved one, and them to you.

Central Need 4—Grieve your losses
As a dementia care partner, you will grieve and mourn for your loved one with dementia just as someone would who experiences loss

through death. The kinds of losses you will endure include personal losses, relationship losses, and the loss of peace of mind. The grief and loss experience will also impact your entire family.

Central Need 5—Take care of yourself
Being a dementia care partner stresses you physically, emotionally, and spiritually, placing you at greater risk for medical problems, depression and anxiety, and social isolation. Being intentional about self-care and wellness will give you the strength and endurance needed for the long journey of dementia caregiving.

Central Need 6—Ask for and accept help from others
Caregiving is a team sport. Most care partners try to do too much themselves and are reluctant to ask for and accept the help of others. It's OK to ask for help! Being intentional about forming a care team will help your loved one receive the best care possible and reduce the burden you experience providing for them.

Central Need 7—Prepare for what's ahead
As your loved one transitions into the later stage of dementia, hard-to-manage behaviors and other changes and challenges require that you get more help at home or even consider full-time residential care. Being proactive about care needs and related legal and financial issues allows you to navigate the journey with less stress.

Central Need 8—Explore existential and spiritual questions to find meaning
Inevitably, when you or someone you love develops a terrible disease like dementia, you often ask questions like "Why him?" or "Why her?" It is important that you feel the freedom to ask such questions, even if they're unanswerable, to help you find meaning and purpose in what otherwise seems senseless.

Symptoms of the Four Most Common Forms of Dementia

APPENDIX 6

Alzheimer's Disease

The "4 A's"

☐ Amnesia – short-term memory loss

☐ Aphasia – difficulty speaking or understanding language

☐ Agnosia – trouble recognizing familiar objects and/or people

☐ Apraxia – impaired purposeful movement like using a fork and knife to eat

Other symptoms

☐ Difficulty multitasking, organizing and planning, and problem-solving

☐ Poor judgment, such as with financial matters

☐ Spatial function challenges, such as getting lost while driving, difficulty navigating stairs or curbs, and falling

☐ Changes in mood, usually depression and often anxiety

☐ Personality changes (social withdrawal, suspicion, or even paranoia), delusions (believing something that isn't true, such as infidelity or theft), obsessive/compulsive tendencies, and doing/saying inappropriate things

Vascular Dementia

Any symptoms listed above for Alzheimer's disease, plus one or more of the following:

- ☐ Drooping or numbness on one side of the face
- ☐ Weakness in an arm and/or leg on one side of the body
- ☐ Speech difficulties (not understanding what is being said, or spoken words not coming out correctly)
- ☐ Impaired vision

Behavioral Variant Frontotemporal Dementia

- ☐ Socially inappropriate behavior in conjunction with poor judgment, such as saying or doing things, even to strangers, that are considered unacceptable (sexually-oriented comments, inappropriate touch, poor manners, and reckless behavior without regard to consequences)
- ☐ Lack of initiative or motivation (apathy)
- ☐ Loss of sympathy and empathy
- ☐ Development of obsessive, repetitive, and/or ritualistic behaviors or speech
- ☐ Carbohydrate craving, especially candies, cookies, and desserts
- ☐ Binge eating, drinking, and/or smoking
- ☐ Loss of insight
- ☐ Difficulty planning, problem-solving, and multitasking

Note: memory is usually normal, especially in the early stage of the disease

Lewy Body Dementia

☐ **Cognitive:** impaired attention span and/or judgment (but insight usually normal), and impaired spatial function and balance (increased fall risk). Short-term memory may or may not be impaired.

☐ **Physical:** slowness of movement, especially walking; shuffles feet while walking; often hunched over and looking down; unsteadiness with frequent falls, tremulousness of the hands; blank expression on face (also referred to as facial masking); and muscle stiffness or rigidity. Later in the disease, loss of the gag reflex and aspiration (inadvertently swallowing liquids or solids into the lungs, choking and pneumonia) can occur.

☐ **Behavioral:** apathy; depression; delusions; hallucinations (seeing things that aren't there, sometimes hearing things too, which may or may not be frightening); nightmares (aggressive acting out of dreams or nightmares, referred to as rapid eye movement or REM sleep disorder); and compulsive behaviors (such as repetitively taking things apart and putting them back together)

☐ **Autonomic:** body-temperature changes (feels hot and sweaty or cold and shivering); irregularities of blood pressure (usually too low, with dizziness or fainting); irregularities in heart and breathing rates (usually too fast, may include a heart condition called atrial fibrillation); digestive issues (bloating or indigestion); bladder or bowel problems (difficulty urinating, frequent urination at night, urgency to go, incontinence); impotence; and a decreased or fluctuating level of alertness and wakefulness

☐ **Other:** rapid cycling of good and bad days

Understanding Our Emotions Exercise

APPENDIX 7

For this activity, circle the emotions you feel the most right now, then choose one and only one among those circled, and write it in the space provided below. Then write down why you chose this emotion. You'll be sharing this with the group. See a list of emotions on the next page that may help you get started.

More than anything else, right now I feel _____

_____

_____

because_____

_____

_____

_____

_____

_____

_____.

Here's the list of emotions you can choose from:

Abandoned	Fragmented	Regretful
Afraid	Frantic	Relieved
Angry	Frightened	Resentful
Anxious	Frustrated	Sad
Ashamed	Furious	Scared
Betrayed	Grief-stricken	Shameful
Bewildered	Guilty	Shocked
Bitter	Happy	Stunned
Confused	Hateful	Surprised
Crazy	Heartbroken	Terrified
Crushed	Helpless	Terrorized
Defeated	Hopeless	Trapped
Depressed	Horrified	Unwanted
Desolate	Hurt	Weak
Desperate	Irritable	Worried
Devastated	Jealous	Worthless
Disbelieving	Joyful	Yearnful
Disgusted	Lonely	Zoned Out
Disorganized	Lost	
Distraught	Loveless	
Embarrassed	Mad	
Empty	Numb	
Encouraged	OK	
Envious	Overwhelmed	
Fearful	Panicked	
Fed Up	Powerless	
Flustered	Rageful	

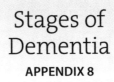

Stages of
Dementia
APPENDIX 8

For the Stages of Dementia, place a checkmark next to any symptoms you have observed in your loved one or that describe their current status.

Mild Cognitive Impairment

☐ Repeats questions or stories

☐ Loses their train of thought

☐ Enters a room but forgets why

☐ Misplaces keys

☐ Has had a noticeable change in performance at work or home (less focused, more disorganized, indecisive, and easily overwhelmed).

☐ MMSE score 25-27; MoCA score 18-25 (see page 81 in *The Dementia Care-Partner's Workbook*)

☐ Independent in instrumental and basic ADLs

☐ Personality and mood normal or "a little off" (spacy, moody, irritable, not themselves)

☐ Orientation normal (knows day, date, month, year, where they are, and where they live)

Early Stage

- [ ] Frequently repeat questions and stories, forgets recent conversations or events, and frequently misplaces things (most true with Alzheimer's; less so with other dementias)
- [ ] Has difficulty with cooking, house cleaning and laundry, getting bills paid on time and/or correctly, and taking pills properly or remembering them at all
- [ ] Gets lost while driving, especially to unfamiliar places
- [ ] Is disorganized when grocery shopping and forget items, even with a list
- [ ] Experiences difficulty finding the right word at times
- [ ] Has trouble planning, problem-solving, and multitasking to the degree that this is very apparent, both at work and at home
- [ ] MMSE score 20-24; MoCA score 11-17
- [ ] May need assistance in some instrumental ADLs; independent in basic ADLs
- [ ] Changes in personality and/or mood are evident (decreased concentration, more irritable and moody, overt depression and/or anxiety, less interest in socializing, activities, and trying new things, may deny there is anything wrong with them)
- [ ] Orientation (knowing day, date, month, season, year, where they live) is normal or a little fuzzy (may be slightly off in day or date, knows rest)

Middle Stage

☐ Repeats questions over and over, shows little interest in or recall of current and recent events, and cannot remember their personal details (such as address and phone number)

☐ Recalls long-term memories (such as knowing their own name and remembering some childhood memories), but they may no longer recognize grandchildren and infrequently seen family or friends

☐ Is unable to cook, clean house, pay bills, take medication, or drive

☐ Requires some assistance in picking out clothes as well as requires a reminder to change clothes (and underwear) daily, usually still able to dress themselves

☐ Goes to the toilet on their own, but hygiene may be poor. Might experience occasional episodes of incontinence, may need reminders and possibly some assistance bathing or showering (may resist hygiene) and might require some help eating (for example, cutting meat)

☐ May require assistance getting out of bed or up from a chair

☐ Expressing themselves verbally may be difficult

☐ Seems apathetic and unmotivated, experiences afternoon and evening confusion and agitation, may be paranoid (about infidelity and theft), experiences delusions and hallucinations, and exhibits obsessive thoughts and compulsive repetitive behaviors

☐ Sleeps up to 12 hours a day but can have long stretches without sleep if agitated. Normal sleep patterns may be disrupted (such as being awake during the night and sleeping during the day).

☐ Requires assistance then becomes dependent in all instrumental ADLs; at end of middle stage will start needing help with basic ADLs (getting dressed is usually first)

☐ MMSE score13-20; MoCA score 6-10

☐ Personality and/or mood changes likely very apparent (person is apathetic and unmotivated, even withdrawn and socially isolated, may have little to no insight into their condition, stay very close to loved ones as if "velcroed at the hip")

☐ Has confusion and disorientation to the day, date, month, and/or year

Late Stage

☐ Unable to cook, clean, do laundry, shop, pay bills, take medicine on their own, use the phone, or drive (dependent in all instrumental ADLs)

☐ Needs progressively more help and eventually requires full assistance getting dressed, showering, going to the bathroom, eating, and getting up from bed or a chair (dependent in all basic ADLs)

☐ Incontinent

☐ Is mostly unaware of and unresponsive to their surroundings

☐ Unable to talk intelligibly, walk, or swallow by the end

☐ MMSE score <12; MoCA score <5 (may not even be able to take test)

☐ Confused and disoriented

Which stage best describes your loved one's current status—MCI, early-middle-, or late-stage dementia? _____

_____

_____

_____

_____

_____

_____

_____

_____

_____

_____

_____

_____

_____

_____

_____

_____

_____

_____

_____

Wellness Wheel and Wellness Plan

APPENDIX 9

Taking care of each dimension of the Wellness Wheel can help you become more aware of the interconnectedness of each dimension, and how all aspects of your life contribute to feeling well, both physically and mentally. Find the Wellness Wheel diagram on the next page.

SPIRITUAL — Find meaning in life events, demonstrate individual purpose, and live a life that reflects your values and beliefs.

EMOTIONAL — Have a positive attitude, high self-esteem, a strong sense of self, and the ability to recognize and share a wide range of feelings with others in a constructive way.

ENVIRONMENTAL — Be aware of the interactions between the environment, community, and yourself, and behave in ways that care for each of these responsibly.

FINANCIAL — Live within your means and learn to manage your finances for the short- and long- term.

SOCIAL — Build personal relationships with others, deal with conflict appropriately, and connect in a positive social network.

PHYSICAL — Take care of your body for optimal health and function.

OCCUPATIONAL — Seek to have a career that is interesting, enjoyable, meaningful, and that contributes to the larger society.

INTELLECTUAL — Be open to new ideas, be creative, think critically, and seek out new challenges.

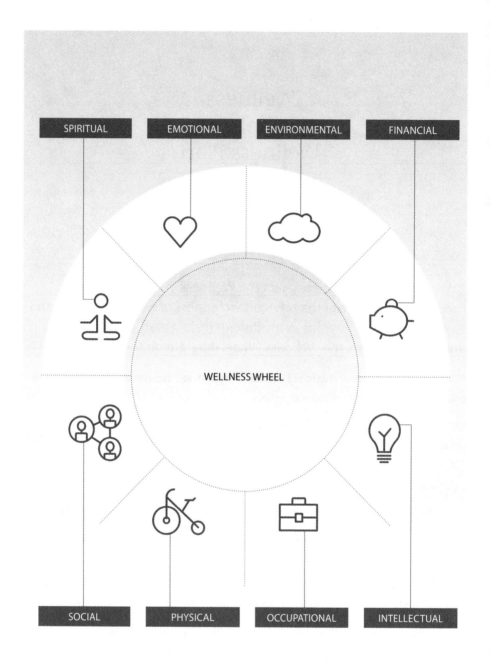

WELLNESS WHEEL

SPIRITUAL

EMOTIONAL

ENVIRONMENTAL

FINANCIAL

SOCIAL

PHYSICAL

OCCUPATIONAL

INTELLECTUAL

Modified from University of New Hampshire Health & Wellness website: https://www.unh.edu/health/well/wellness

A Leader's Manual for Dementia Care-Partner Support Groups

I, _____, commit to doing the following
(your name here)

for the next month because my wellness is important to me,

_____, and my family.
(name of your loved one with dementia)

1. To improve my physical health, I will _____
   _____
   _____

2. To improve my mental health, I will _____
   _____
   _____

3. To improve my social relationships, I will _____
   _____
   _____

4. To improve my spiritual health, I will _____
   _____
   _____

At the end of one month, I will reevaluate.

Signed: _____

Date:_____

Support-Group Participant Evaluation Form

APPENDIX 10

Please answer the following questions related to the support group you just completed. Thank you!

I help care for someone who has (check one):

☐ Alzheimer's disease

☐ Vascular dementia

☐ Behavioral variant frontotemporal dementia

☐ Primary progressive aphasia or another form of dementia mainly affecting speech and language

☐ Lewy body dementia or dementia associated with Parkinson's disease

☐ Another form of dementia
  Please name:_____

1. How did you find out about this group?

  ☐ From my doctor or medical provider

  ☐ From my counselor or mental-healthcare provider

  ☐ Friend/word-of-mouth

  ☐ A community agency:_____

  ☐ My retirement community:_____

  ☐ Flyer

  ☐ Newspaper ad

  ☐ Other. Please specify: _____

2. What did you hope to gain from the group? Check all that apply and circle the one that was your most important reason.

  ☐ To learn more about memory loss or dementia

  ☐ To learn more about how to care for a loved one with memory loss or dementia

  ☐ To meet other people who are dealing with memory loss or dementia

  ☐ To have an opportunity to talk about my challenges

  ☐ Other. Please specify: _____

3. Did the group you attended meet your expectations? Circle one response.

  Not at all   1   2   3   4   5   Very much

4. What do you think was the MOST HELPFUL aspect of the group?

_____

_____

_____

_____

_____

_____

5. What do you think was the LEAST HELPFUL aspect of the group?

_____

_____

_____

_____

_____

_____

6. On a scale of 1–5, how would you rate your knowledge of memory loss or dementia BEFORE attending this group? Circle one response.

Not at all knowledgeable   1   2   3   4   5   Very knowledgeable

7. On a scale of 1–5, how would you rate your knowledge of memory loss or dementia AFTER attending this group? Circle one response.

Not at all knowledgeable   1   2   3   4   5   Very knowledgeable

8. On a scale of 1–5, how would you rate your coping skills BEFORE attending this group? Circle one response.

Not coping well   1   2   3   4   5   Coping very well

9. On a scale of 1–5, how would you rate your coping skills AFTER attending this group? Circle one response.

Not coping well   1   2   3   4   5   Coping very well

10. Please answer the following questions about the leader(s) who facilitated the group. Circle one response for each question.

Were knowledgeable about memory loss or dementia	Yes	No	Not sure/NA
Were compassionate	Yes	No	Not sure/NA
Helped me to feel safe and accepted in the setting I was in	Yes	No	Not sure/NA
Helped me to develop skills for dealing with memory loss or dementia	Yes	No	Not sure/NA
Offered information about additional resources	Yes	No	Not sure/NA
Managed the group dynamics well	Yes	No	Not sure/NA
Provided opportunities for me to ask questions, contribute, and/or share	Yes	No	Not sure/NA
Provided opportunities for us/all present to contribute, and/or share	Yes	No	Not sure/NA

11. After participating in this group, would you recommend it to a friend or family member living with or caring for someone with memory loss or dementia? Circle one response.

Not at all   1   2   3   4   5   Very likely

12. How could we improve this group?

_____

_____

_____

_____

_____

_____

13. Ideas for other groups?

_____

_____

_____

_____

_____

_____

14. Other comments and suggestions?

_____

_____

_____

_____

_____

Resources For Support-Group Members

APPENDIX 11

BOOKS

- *Keeping Love Alive as Memories Fade: The 5 Love Languages and the Alzheimer's Journey.* Deborah Barr, Edward G. Shaw, and Gary Chapman. 2016.

- *The 36-Hour Day.* Nancy L. Mace and Peter V. Rabins. 6th edition. 2017.

- *The Alzheimer's Action Plan: What You Need to Know—and What You Can Do—About Memory Problems, from Prevention to Early Intervention and Care.* P. Murali Doraiswamy and Lisa P. Gwyther. 2009.

- *Creating Moments of Joy Along the Alzheimer's Journey: A Guide for Families and Caregivers.* Jolene Brackey. 5th Edition. 2008

- *Healing Your Grieving Heart When Someone You Care About Has Alzheimer's: 100 Practical Ideas for Families, Friends, and Caregivers.* Alan D. Wolfelt and Kirby J. Duvall. 2011.

- *Grace for the Unexpected Journey: A 60-Day Devotional for Alzheimer's and Other Dementia Caregivers.* Deborah Barr. 2018.

DEMENTIA EDUCATIONAL PRODUCTS, PODCASTS, AND TED TALKS

- Teepa Snow and the Positive Approach to Care: **www.teepasnow.com**

- The Fight Against Alzheimer's and Dementia (TED Talk, Samuel Cohen): https://www.ted.com/playlists/443/the_fight_against_alzheimer_s
- Johns Hopkins Medical Podcasts on Alzheimer's and Dementia: https://podcasts.hopkinsmedicine.org/category/podcasts/healthtopics/alzheimers-disease-and-dementia/
- Embodied Labs Virtual Reality Training for Alzheimer's Disease and Lewy Body Dementia: www.embodiedlabs.com

MINDFULNESS

- *Mindfulness for Beginners: Reclaiming the Present Moment for Your Life.* Jon Kabat-Zinn. Sounds True, Boulder, CO, 2016.
- *Wherever You Go, There You Are: Mindfulness Meditation in Everyday Life.* Jon Kabat-Zinn, Hyperion, New York, NY, 2005.
- *Dancing With Elephants: Mindfulness Training for Those Living With Dementia, Chronic Illness or an Aging Brain.* Jarem Sawatsky. 2017.
- Apps: Mindfulness Daily (www.mindfulnessdailyapp.com) and Aura (www.aurahealth.io).

OTHER

- Powerful Tools for Caregivers: www.powerfultoolsforcaregivers.org

WEBSITES

- The Alzheimer's Association: www.alz.org
- The Alzheimer's Foundation of America: www.alzfdn.org
- The Dementia Action Alliance: www.daanow.org
- African Americans Against Alzheimer's: www.usagainstalzheimers.org

- Alzheimer's Disease International:
  www.alz.co.uk
- Lewy Body Dementia Association:
  www.lbda.org
- The Association for Frontotemporal Degeneration:
  www.theaftd.org
- The National Institute on Aging:
  www.nia.nih.gov
- The National Institute of Neurologic Disorders and Stroke:
  www.ninds.nih.gov

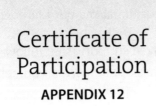

Certificate of
Participation

*Use this template to create a Certificate of Participation" for your group
members.*

**CERTIFICATE OF DEMENTIA CARE-PARTNER SUPPORT GROUP
PARTICIPATION**

Be it known that on this day:

_____

has completed *The Dementia Care-Partner's Workbook* support group,
learned about and internalized the following eight central needs of
dementia care partners, and gained understanding, education, and
hope to continue on the journey caring for a loved one with dementia.

Central Need 1—Tell and retell your story

Central Need 2—Educate yourself

Central Need 3—Adapt to changing relationships

Central Need 4—Grieve your losses

Central Need 5—Take care of yourself

Central Need 6—Ask for and accept help from others

Central Need 7—Prepare for what's ahead

Central Need 8—Explore existential and spiritual questions to find meaning

You have given and received support from fellow group members, learned how to be compassionate toward yourself, and made a personal commitment to wellness. For your participation, care, compassion, concern, and love, we are grateful. We wish you continued strength and renewed hope each and every day on the journey down a path not chosen.

_____

Group Leader(s)

_____

_____

_____

Date

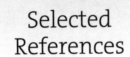

Selected
References

Samuel T. Gladding. *Groups: A Counseling Specialty* (6th Edition, 2011). Merrill Counseling.

Alan D. Wolfelt. *The Understanding Your Grief Support Group Guide: Starting and Leading a Bereavement Support Group*, 2004. Companion Press.

Alan D. Wolfelt. *The Understanding Your Suicide Grief Support Group Guide: Meeting Plans for Facilitators*, 2010. Companion Press.

Alan D. Wolfelt. *Counseling Skills for Companioning the Mourner: The Fundamentals of Effective Grief Counseling*, 2016. Companion Press.

Feedback

To the support group leaders who have used the *Leader's Manual*, thank you for the time you've committed and the compassion you've shown to the dementia care partners you've companioned through *The Dementia Care-Partner's Workbook* and this *Leader's Manual*. I would love your feedback! Here are a few suggested questions to guide your response, or feel free to provide comments and suggestions however you see fit. Please email your thoughts to me at drshaw@ empatheducation.com. Thanks so much!

1. What did you find most helpful about the *Leader's Manual*?

2. What did you find least helpful about the *Leader's Manual*?

3. What additions would you suggest to make the *Leader's Manual* more helpful?

4. What other support-group materials would you find useful to support care partners or those with dementia?

5. Tell me a bit about yourself, and, if appropriate, the organization you work for.

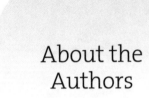

About the Authors

EDWARD G. SHAW, M.D., M.A.

Edward G. Shaw, M.D., M.A., is dually trained as a physician and mental-health counselor. He was the primary care partner for his late wife, Rebecca, who was diagnosed with early-onset Alzheimer's disease in 2008, at age 53. She died in 2016 after a nine-year battle. He was a practicing academic radiation oncologist for 23 years, specializing in the treatment of adults and children with brain cancer. In 2010, inspired by Rebecca's journey, he found that his medical interest shifted to dementia diagnosis and treatment, and after additional training in mental-health counseling, he founded the Memory Counseling Program in 2011, part of Gerontology and Geriatric Medicine and the Sticht Center for Healthy Aging and Alzheimer's Prevention at Wake Forest Baptist Health, in Winston-Salem, North Carolina. The program serves individuals, couples, and families affected by Alzheimer's disease or another form of dementia. Ed is founder of Empath Education, a company whose mission is to provide empathy-based education to people with dementia, their care partners, and medical and mental-healthcare professionals who work with older adults, including those affected by Alzheimer's disease or another form of dementia. He is author of the newly released book *The Dementia Care-Partner's Workbook*, a support-group curriculum or self-study manual for family care partners who have a loved one with Alzheimer's disease or another form of dementia. With Ms. Deborah Barr and Dr. Gary Chapman, he co-authored the book *Keeping Love Alive as Memories Fade: The 5 Love Languages and the Alzheimer's Journey* in 2016, which describes his moving personal story of caring for Rebecca coupled with an innovative use of the five love languages in dementia counseling and care. Ed resides in Winston-Salem with his wife, Claire. He has three adult daughters, Erin, Leah, and Carrie, a son-in-law, Darian, two grandsons, Paul and Isaiah, and a stepson, Patrick.

ALAN D. WOLFELT, PH.D.

Alan D. Wolfelt, Ph.D., is an internationally noted author, educator, and grief counselor. Known for his model of "companioning" versus "treating" mourners, Dr. Wolfelt has become a "responsible rebel" who advocates for grief care that is compassionate, griever-led, and soul-and-spirit-based.

He is the author of a number of bestselling books on grief and loss. Among his titles are *Companioning the Bereaved, Understanding Your Grief,* and *Healing Your Grieving Heart When Someone You Care About Has Alzheimer's.* Past recipient of the Association of Death Education and Counseling's Death Educator Award, Dr. Wolfelt also serves as the Director of the Center for Loss and Life Transition and is on the faculty at the University of Colorado Medical School's Department of Family Medicine.

To contact
Dr. Shaw or
Dr. Wolfelt

To contact Dr. Shaw about speaking engagements, training opportunities, or consulting for your organization, visit his website www.empatheducation.com or email him at drshaw@empatheducation.com.

To contact Dr. Wolfelt about speaking engagements or training opportunities at the Center for Loss and Life Transition, visit www.centerforloss.com, call (970) 226-6050 or email him at DrWolfelt@centerforloss.com.

Downloadable
Version!

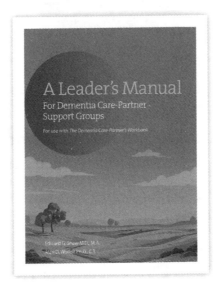

A Leader's Manual
For Dementia Care-Partner
Support Groups

For use with *The Dementia Care-Partner's Workbook*

Edward G. Shaw MD, M.A.
Alan D. Wolfelt Ph.D., C.T.

This book is available as a downloadable PDF!
Simply purchase the PDF online and download instantly.

Sized at 8.5x11 so you can print out individual sheets as needed.

$19.95 • 113 pages • 8.5x11

Available at: www.centerforloss.com/bookstore/dementia-leaders-manual

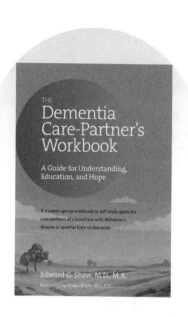

The Dementia Care-Partner's Workbook:
A Guide for Understanding, Education, and Hope

By Edward G. Shaw, M.D., M.A.

The Dementia Care-Partner's Workbook is a support group manual as well as a self-study guide for care partners of a loved one with Alzheimer's disease or another type of dementia. It provides 13 lessons for support group participants or individuals who desire independent study.

The Dementia Care-Partner's Workbook is authored by Dr. Edward Shaw, a dually trained physician and mental health counselor who directs a large dementia caregiver support program and is an experienced support group leader. He was also care partner to his late wife Rebecca, who lost her nine year battle with Alzheimer's disease several years ago.

ISBN 978-1-61722-274-0 • 290 pages • softcover • $19.95

Available at: www.centerforloss.com/bookstore

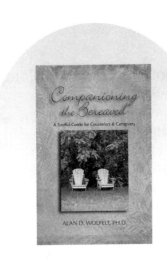

Companioning the Bereaved
A Soulful Guide for Caregivers

This book by one of North America's most respected grief educators presents a model for grief counseling based on his "companioning" principles.

For many mental healthcare providers, grief in contemporary society has been medicalized— perceived as if it were an illness that with proper assessment, diagnosis, and treatment could be cured.

Dr. Wolfelt explains that our modern understanding of grief all too often conveys that at bereavement's "end" the mourner has completed a series of tasks, extinguished pain, and established new relationships. Our psychological models emphasize "recovery" or "resolution" in grief, suggesting a return to "normalcy."

By contrast, this book advocates a model of "companioning" the bereaved, acknowledging that grief forever changes or transforms the mourner's world view. Companioning is not about assessing, analyzing, fixing, or resolving another's grief. Instead, it is about being totally present to the mourner, even being a temporary guardian of his soul.

ISBN 978-1-879651-41-8 • 191 pages • hardcover • $29.95

Available at: www.centerforloss.com/bookstore

Other Support Group Guides from Companion Press

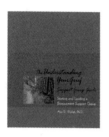

The Understanding Your Grief Support Group Guide
STARTING AND LEADING A BEREAVEMENT SUPPORT GROUP

For bereavement caregivers who want to start and run an effective grief support group for adults, this support group guide discusses the role of support groups for mourners and describes the steps involved (such as deciding on group format, publicizing the group, and writing meeting plans) in getting a group started. Responding to problems in the group is also addressed, as is a model for evaluating your group's progress.

This guide includes potential meeting plans that interface with Understanding Your Grief and the companion journal as texts for group participants. This support group guide is a must for all bereavement group leaders.

ISBN 978-1-879651-40-1 • 104 pages • softcover • $19.95

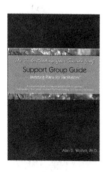

The Understanding Your Suicide Grief Support Group Guide
MEETING PLANS FOR FACILITATORS

This book is for those who want to facilitate an effective suicide grief support group. It includes 12 meeting plans that interface with Understanding Your Suicide Grief and its companion journal.

ISBN 978-1-879651-60-9 • 52 pages • softcover • $12.95

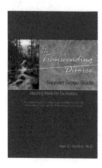

The Transcending Divorce Support Group Guide
MEETING PLANS FOR FACILITATORS

This book is for those who want to facilitate an effective divorce group. It includes 12 meeting plans that interface with Dr. Wolfelt's Transcending Divorce book and its companion journal.

ISBN 978-1-879651-56-2 • 52 pages • softcover • $12.95

Available at: www.centerforloss.com/bookstore